Welcome to the YOPD Club

WILLIAM J BRADDOCK

WELCOME TO THE YOPD CLUB

DEDICATION

I would like to dedicate this book to the roughly 4% of people who are diagnosed with Young Onset Parkinson's Disease (YOPD) each year. We are part of the "Parkinson's Pandemic" which accounts for 7-10% of people worldwide. I would also like to dedicate this book to the people featured in these chapters who shared their time, experience and wisdom with me. Without your honesty and sharing, this book would not have been possible.

WELCOME TO THE YOPD CLUB

CONTENTS

Medical Terms	1
Forward	7
Chapter 1: My Story	17
Chapter 2: Jimmy Choi	31
Chapter 3: Larry Gifford	49
Chapter 4: Kristen Gray	67
Chapter 5: Bret Parker	79
Chapter 6: Christina Korines	91
Chapter 7: Gavin Mogan	103
Chapter 8: Heather Kennedy	119
Chapter 9: Paul Cluff	129
Introduction of Paola Celi	139
Chapter 10: Paola Celi	143
Closing Remarks	153
Acknowledgements	159

WELCOME TO THE YOPD CLUB

MEDICAL TERMS

Here is a brief description of all the medical terms that I refer to in this book:

Alpha-Synuclein Protein: A faulty protein that suffocates the brain cells that produce dopamine.

Amantadine: A prescription medication that is prescribed to treat mild symptoms in early Parkinson's Disease, but most often prescribed to treat dyskinesia.

Azilect®: The only FDA approved MAOB inhibitor that can be taken by itself for Parkinson's Disease.

Bradykinesia: Slowness of movement.

Carbidopa-Levadopa (Sinemet aka L-Dopa): The most widely prescribed dopamine replacement therapy drug used to treat Parkinson's Disease. It is absorbed in the intestine and the brain converts it to dopamine. Long term usage can lead to dyskinesia.

Citalopram®: A prescription medication used to treat depression. It works by helping to restore the balance of serotonin in the brain.

DAT Scan: An imaging test used to help diagnose Parkinson's Disease.

Deep Brain Stimulation: This is a neurological procedure involving the installation of a neurotransmitter that sends electrical impulses to specific targets in the brain. This procedure is recommended for people with symptoms that can not be adequately controlled with medication.

Dopamine: A chemical in the brain that coordinates movement but decreases in Parkinson's Disease.

Dopamine Agonist: Medications that mimic the effect of dopamine. In some people, these drugs can lead to impulse control disorders.

Dyskinesia: Uncontrolled involuntary writhing or wriggling movements. It most often occurs when symptoms are otherwise well-controlled (known as "on times").

Dystonia: A movement disorder in which a person's muscles

MEDICAL TERMS

contract uncontrollably. It can affect one muscle, a muscle group, or the entire body.

Glial Derived Neurotrophic Factor (GDNF): A groundbreaking trial involved implanting a novel delivery system into the brain to infuse a protein periodically in a clinical setting and involved 42 participants. The protein named Glial Derived Neurotrophic Factor was to be checked for disease-modifying capability. It is well documented that there was a huge gap between the scientific findings and the patient experience from receiving GDNF.

INBRIJA®: Levodopa that is inhaled through your mouth to help treat the return of Parkinson's symptoms between regular doses of medication.

Lexapro®: A prescription medication that is used to treat the symptoms of major depressive disorder and generalized anxiety disorder.

MAOB Inhibitors: These medications block an enzyme in the brain that breaks down dopamine after it does its work. They allow the available dopamine to function for a longer period-of-time.

Mirapex®: A dopamine agonist that can improve the ability to move and decrease shakiness.

Movement Disorder Specialist: A neurologist with

additional training in Parkinson's Disease and other movement disorders.

Neuro Patch: A patch that is worn on the skin that delivers the dopamine agonist, Rotigotine, directly into the bloodstream. It releases the medicine 24 hours a day, providing a stable, continuous delivery.

Primidone: A prescription medication that is used to control certain types of seizures. It is in a class of medications called anticonvulsants and works by decreasing abnormal electrical activity in the brain.

Propanolol: A prescription medication that belongs to a group of medicines called beta-blockers. It is used to treat heart problems, help with anxiety, and prevent migraines.

Requip®: A prescription medication that has some of the same effects as dopamine. It is used to treat symptoms such as stiffness, tremors, muscle spasms, and poor muscle control. It is also used to treat restless leg syndrome.

RYTARY®: A controlled release form of Carbidopa-Levodopa.

Synthetic Dopamine: Dopamine that is generated synthetically by way of certain medications.

Unified Parkinson's Disease Rating Scale: A rating tool used to gauge the course of Parkinson's Disease in patients. A

MEDICAL TERMS

score of 199 represents total disability.

Xadago: An MAOP inhibitor that treats "off times" which typically appear in the middle or later phases of Parkinson's Disease. It is an option to be taken several years into the course of the disease.

WELCOME TO THE YOPD CLUB

FORWARD

Parkinson's Disease (PD) is a progressive nerve disease of the brain that in time leads to a debilitation of a person's motor functions. Over time, the individual with PD loses the ability to produce a chemical called dopamine, leading to the classic symptoms of tremor, stiffness, slowness and loss of balance. Most people with PD are diagnosed in their fifties or later. However, it is not just a disease of the elderly. Up to 10% of those with the condition develop the disease in their forties or younger at which point it is termed "Young Onset Parkinson's Disease" (YOPD). According to the researchers behind the book "Ending Parkinson's Disease, A Prescription for Action," beginning in a person's forties, the risk of PD roughly triples with each passing decade. In 2019 alone, 60,000 individuals, or over 1,000 Americans per week, were diagnosed with PD. By 2030, there will be a 10% higher risk of a forty-five-year-old individual eventually developing PD than there is today and with increasing longevity, more of us will face PD. By 2040, the number will double again to at least 12.9 million.

Tim Hague was diagnosed with YOPD at the age of 46 and shortly thereafter, he and his son competed and won the first Amazing Race Canada in 2013. He was the first person with PD to compete in the race and is an inspiration for many as a living, breathing example of what it looks like to overcome adversity. He is also the author of the book "Perseverance, The Seven Skills You Need to Survive, Thrive, and Accomplish More Than You Ever Imagined" and a Parkinson's advocate who lives in Winnipeg, Canada.

I asked Tim to be a contributing author for this book by writing a letter to his newly diagnosed 46-year-old self because his perspective from a 10-year span paints a remarkable picture of what one person's experience living with YOPD looks like. As raw and unapologetic as his perspective is, it is also a reminder that everyone's journey is different. Our symptoms are different, the pace with which the disease progresses is different, our response to medication is different and our sensitivities to our body's changes are different. What does this mean? It means that one person's story will greatly differ from another's and as a newly diagnosed Person with Parkinson's (PWP), there is no sense in comparing journeys because we're all dealing with the disease at our own pace and tolerance.

Tim, if you could write a letter to your newly diagnosed 46-year-old self knowing then what you know now, what would you say to him?

You're screwed.

Okay, maybe that's not the way I would start the conversation, but it would be very tempting. That is an awfully tough way to start a conversation though. Furthermore, it may not be true for you as a person newly diagnosed with Parkinson's disease. But, then again it may be. In almost ten years with Parkinson's disease my experience is that we as a community tend to gloss over our more difficult realities. We don't like to go to the really hard places of this disease. I know that I have wanted to focus on hope, encouragement and exercise and while the importance of these have not changed, I have come to see another need. That need is the awareness, a warning, that some do die from this disease and it can be so much more difficult than 'just a tremor'.

I knew it or at least I had a sense of it. I had seen my father live out his last years with Parkinson's as one of his many ailments. I had nursed many others with this disease. But you don't ever know a thing until you have lived with it for a time. These many years later there are a number of things I would go back and tell my 46-year-old self if I could.

    I would tell myself that this disease is horrible and the younger you are when you get it the longer and potentially worse it will be. For you see it won't kill you; at least not quickly. It will let you live while it tears strips off your life, steals your abilities and attempts to crush your dreams. You will be told over and again that Parkinson's does not define your life, yet, for most, it will come to set the rules of your every waking hour not to mention many of those in which you try to sleep. You will see spouses broken and marriages shattered; the fittest of individuals hobbled, rich, productive minds left clouded. You will witness the buckling of brave souls beneath the weight of an unrelenting foe.

    These are the things we are seldom told or are said quietly in passing on our way to the 'you can do this' cheering section.

    It may be that none of these things will ever apply to you, but then again, they may. They certainly apply to many who struggle with PD.

    I understand that this is likely not what you want to read. You would likely be far happier with my book, "Perseverance, The Seven Skills You Need to Survive,

FORWARD

Thrive, and Accomplish More Than You Ever Imagined". It's an inspirational piece guiding you in how-to skills in living your best with Parkinson's. It's totally positive. But...

I would tell myself early on that many are far too cavalier with the positive messages attributed to Parkinson's; these ideas that 'Parkinson's will not define me', 'It's not a death sentence, it is a life sentence' and on and on. Recently, an elder entertainer was diagnosed in his 80's and made the statement that, 'this PD thing is no big deal'. I was angry.

Angry because of an attitude that did not take the time to know my friends whose lives have been brought low by Parkinson's. Those in their 30's, 40's, and 50's whose bodies will no longer heed their commands. Limbs that flail or that will not move at all. Guts that will not absorb nutrients and slowly starve their bodies. Bodies that simply refuse to accept most medications. Those who function at all only due to a miracle surgical procedure where electrodes are placed in one's brain. Those living with all this while attempting to raise children and keep marriages and their lives together. No, this PD thing is no big deal. It can be a nightmare.

I would tell my 46-year-old self that you must hear

the whole truth in the statements made about Parkinson's. For example; 'Parkinson's is typically a slow moving, or progressing, disease'. This is great news unless you ask the question, 'compared to what?' compared to a cancer like pancreatic cancer which tends to be a death sentence then, yes, PD is great news. However, few ever really explain what the 'slow moving' will look like or do to you. If you are diagnosed at say 46 and you get a solid ten to fifteen years out of life, that means that you are between fifty-six and sixty-one when you run out of "solid years"! A reasonably young person still pre-retirement age but none the less worn out by the drip, drip, drip of a chronic and progressive disease that is "slow moving".

Our community, like much of society, can find it difficult to talk about mental health. Yet more than 50 percent of us will suffer with depression, anxiety and various psychological concerns. That's a big number. I would have told my newly diagnosed self to add a psychologist to my healthcare team sooner, from the beginning.

There are many other things I would add to the list of advice and warnings that I would have given myself some ten years ago:

FORWARD

Don't quit your job too soon. Freedom 51, or my play on the old insurance commercial 'Freedom 55', is not fun.

Start your meds (Carbidopa-Levodopa) sooner. Had I done so I am convinced I would have gotten another few years out of my job. For the guy who never really enjoyed going to work every day it has been much more difficult not being able to go to my chosen profession every day. Had I started the meds sooner I believe I would have had an all-around better quality of life in my early years.

Don't ever stop running. Don't ever stop cycling. Exercise...more. Running and cycling have been my outlets for exercise. Whatever yours are, don't stop doing them. As a matter of fact, do more. This is one measure of control that you can retain in positively impacting your symptoms.

Travel more. That is have fun, enjoy life. Whatever it is that you like to do, do more. There is a hard stop coming, a day when you will not be able to do some of the things you want to do. Do them now.

Be joyful. Be content. Practice perseverance. Give hope. I would tell my 46-year-old self that this disease is different for everyone and that my journey, has thus far, been easier than most. Yet, even then most of the others will be happy, joyful, content; they will stay on their journey and offer me hope. I would tell myself that no matter how dark my days get there are those living darker lives. Be grateful, offer hope.

I would tell my 46-year-old, newly diagnosed self, amid attempting to understand and respond to the whole of the disease not to lose focus...don't lose hope. I would remind myself that only through embracing our suffering do we learn to persevere, that through perseverance our character is deepened, and through this change in character we discover hope. There is no hope without first embracing the suffering.

...

FORWARD

This book is written primarily for the newly diagnosed Young Onset Person with Parkinson's (YOPWP), but it's also for the care givers, family members, friends and associates who like me, are approaching this disease for the first time or with questions about what to expect.

It has been written in the format of a journalistic interview that includes questions from me and answers from 10 inspirational people that are living with YOPD. I have crafted my questions to solicit real information about their personal experiences to paint a picture of what it looks like to live with the disease. As you read this book, my hope is that you'll walk away with a sense of comfort that if you were newly diagnosed, rest assured that you are not alone, you did nothing wrong to deserve your diagnosis, you're part of a bigger family and that with a little perseverance, you can manage this disease and live a quality life for many more years to come. If you are a care giver, a family member, a friend or associate that is coming to this book not knowing much about YOPD, my hope is that you walk away with a better understanding of what it looks like and better yet, that you'll have a newfound understanding of how you can support the Person with Parkinson's (PWP) in your life.

With that, Welcome to the YOPD Club!

WELCOME TO THE YOPD CLUB

CHAPTER 1 / MY STORY

MY STORY

God, help me to be excited to see what's next.

When I was first diagnosed with YOPD on December 31, 2019 at the age of 43, one of the things that I found to comfort my nerves was listening to podcasts on the subject. I listened to everything I could find but the one that moved me was Christian Hageseth's podcast. Chris is a 79-year-old psychiatrist who was diagnosed with PD at the age of 71. He was the first person that I came across who had a ferociously positive outlook on the disease and was also the first person aside from my immediate family members that I told about my diagnosis. To this day, his response to the following question still resonates with me in a positive way. The question was: What advice would you give to a person that's been newly diagnosed with PD?

Chris said: *"I tell them that they've got the best damn progressive neurological disease that they could have. You don't have relapsing MS, or a brain tumor, or a stroke that will leave you speechless. What's good about PD is that you can change the course of it if you really put your mind to it. You may eventually find that you have no impairment from it at all."*

At the time of my initial diagnosis, I knew nothing about PD aside from the fact that it was an old person's disease and that Michael J. Fox and Mohammad Ali had it. I didn't have any immediate family members that had the disease so didn't have any direct experience with PD. I also didn't know if there were other people my age that had it either so Chris's perspective resonated with me because it gave me the thing I desperately needed...hope. I had played sports all my life and was familiar with overcoming adversity, so I needed to hear that it was beatable; maybe not curable, but beatable in order for me to sleep at night.

What was my diagnosis like?

My journey with PD started about 4 years before I was formally diagnosed when I noticed a slight hand tremor while talking with my boss about a project. I'm an architect and these discussions were status quo for my occupation so I just ignored it and filed it away as a stress tick or possibly carpal tunnel associated with age and heavy computer usage. It was akin to an eye twitch or a muscle spasm in that it felt like everyone could see it but, in reality, it was unnoticeable. Whatever it was, it wasn't frequent or debilitating enough for me to be concerned with so I ignored it and figured that I would eventually grow into living with it or it

CHAPTER 1 / MY STORY

would go away. For the most part, I could turn it off when it came on, even joke about it with friends to show that I was comfortable with it, so I felt like I had it under control. I was 38 at the time and wasn't in the best health. I wasn't exercising, had high cholesterol, was raising two kids, was managing a competitive job with multiple deadlines, carrying heavy consumer debt and overall was convinced that this was a stress related tick that had manifested itself as a hand tremor.

My Primary Care Physician (PCP) recommended that I see a neurologist in response to my complaint that I had "a weird hand twitch." When I saw the neurologist, she looked me over, had me walk an imaginary catwalk a few times and after about 20 minutes of dexterity and balance tests, told me that I had a B12 deficiency which was the probable cause of a condition called "Benign Essential Hand Tremor." I had never heard of it but was relieved that it had a name and even more so that it had the word "benign" in front of it. I was cautiously optimistic that it was an isolated case and that I could fix the tremor naturally with improved diet, weight loss, exercise and supplements. She also prescribed a medication to target my increasing levels of anxiety called "Propranolol" with the direction to take it when I needed it. Suffice to say, I left my first neurologist's visit feeling reassured that

> SUFFICE TO SAY, I LEFT MY FIRST NEUROLOGIST'S VISIT FEELING REASSURED THAT NOTHING WAS WRONG AND THAT THE SYMPTOMS WERE TREATABLE, BUT AS I LATER LEARNED, I HAD BEEN MIS-DIAGNOSED.

nothing was wrong and that the symptoms were treatable, but as I later learned, I had been mis diagnosed.

Over the next 4 years, I gradually increased my dosage of Propranolol because my anxiety seemed to be getting worse and tried to interject more exercise and healthy eating into my lifestyle convinced that I could naturally beat the tremor. I took the Propranolol ahead of any anxiety prone situations such as speaking in public, or attendance at events where I might be called upon to give a speech on the fly and for the most part, it worked well to calm my nerves. However, I noticed that my tremor was getting progressively worse and that I was having to increase my dosage to counteract the effects. So, my neurologist asked that I try a Parkinson's medication called "Carbidopa-Levodopa" (L-Dopa) to see if I responded. Although it wasn't a diagnosis, when the words "Parkinson's" came out of his mouth, I was shocked that the disease was being mentioned. I had heard of Parkinson's but considered it a disease of the elderly, certainly not something a 40-year-old would be contending with. Besides that, no one had mentioned PD as a possible cause over the past several years of doctor's visits so I thought that if I had it, someone would have noticed something earlier. Determined to debunk the suspicion, I took the medication irregularly for two months and happily reported that the L-Dopa didn't work.

Over the next few years, I took an assortment of prescription cocktails intended to attack the tremor and my neurology visits transitioned into updates on my response to the

CHAPTER 1 / MY STORY

various medications. After the failed L-Dopa trial, I did a low dosage trial of a drug called "Primidone" which exacerbated the tremor and left me depressed most of the time. I couldn't even finish the trial because it was interfering with my performance at work, so I asked for something else. My neurologist had always told me to do a "test run" of the medications over the weekend to see how I would respond so one Sunday morning after breakfast, I tried a half pill of "Citalopram" to see if it made a difference. After about 10 minutes, I noticed that my hand tremor started to violently shake, and my heart rate was spiking. I couldn't sit still and, in a panic, I was walking up and down the stairs in my house to keep up with my pounding heart rate. I felt as if my heart was going to explode so I lay down in my bed until the effects wore off. Between runs to the toilet to relieve frequent diarrhea urges and shaking in my right foot and hand that could only be controlled by physical restraint, I was a mess and obviously knew the medication wasn't right for me. I went back to the Propranolol since it seemed like the only medication that eased my symptoms.

After that Sunday experience, my tremor became noticeably worse and I began to think about it a lot more. Because I was becoming more self-conscious, I started avoiding friends and family and was having to forcibly hold my hand while talking to prevent it from being a distraction. In addition, I decided to teach myself how to eat with my left hand because my right hand would shake so much that I couldn't trust it to deliver food to my mouth. That was the point where I realized that my symptoms were getting bad and I couldn't control it anymore. Then one day while reviewing blood work with my Primary Care Physician (PCP) and trying to hide my "shaky hand," he recommended that I get a second opinion. Three months later, I was sitting with a Movement Disorder Specialist (MDS) that focused on PD and after an hour of talking and testing I heard the following words: "Mr. Braddock, you've been contending with Parkinson's Disease." Four years after my first neurologist's visit where I was told that I had a benign, treatable condition, my first response was: Can I die from this? My second response was that it must have been a mistake because how could one neurologist who saw my progression for the past 4 years see something completely different than a second neurologist that saw me for 1.5 hours? Whatever the reasons were, I was in denial and left the appointment in a state of shock wondering what it all meant.

The hard thing about the diagnosis for me was that it wasn't part of my life plan and I couldn't fix it. Suddenly, I became distracted with Parkinson's. It prevented me from focusing at work, it robbed me of my joy, and it initially made me feel like my life was hopeless. I hadn't planned for it, so I suddenly found myself in reaction mode trying to understand the gravity of the diagnosis and what it meant. The doctors were so ambiguous about disease progression that I didn't know whether it was something to worry about or not. I didn't feel any different physically but certainly felt broken emotionally. Even to hear the MDS summarize my diagnosis to a research assistant on my way to give blood was

CHAPTER 1 / MY STORY

painful. I had been so excited about the visit because I was convinced that the MDS would dismiss my symptoms as stress related or confirm the essential tremor diagnosis, yet here I was, 9AM on December 31, 2019, having just received a life changing diagnosis. Any attempt to laugh, celebrate, or enjoy New Year's Eve was hollow because I was officially broken. I even questioned the validity of the examination thinking that it was too subjective to be accurate. So, for me, the diagnosis was questionable at best and I didn't want to accept it partly because it was an admission that I was now damaged goods.

The day after my diagnosis, I came downstairs, poured myself a cup of coffee and broke into tears talking to my wife. I realized that I knew nothing about the disease and felt completely vulnerable. I didn't know the life expectancy of the disease, if I'd get to see my kids grow up and get married or have kids of their own. Most of all, I was afraid that my symptoms would prevent me from being able to work, which would force me into early retirement and that I wouldn't be able to afford insurance, or the medication needed to manage the disease. In short, I had my first breakdown.

However, here I am, eight months from formal diagnosis at the time of this writing, but likely 4 years and 6 months into this disease and I have a new perspective. Instead of looking at this disease as a roadblock, I'm excited to see what God has for me next. I've got a quiet confidence, probably developed out of mornings in prayer, that God has a bigger plan for me and it's not for me to understand. The first half of my life was characterized by a fair amount of predictability, but the next will likely be a series of learning experiences and a type of social maturity that I've never prepared for. You know that type of maturity - where you must learn to take yourself less seriously. After all, I'm going to find myself in some humiliating situations, like dropping plates of food at dinner parties because my hand will shake so much. Or having to ask for assistance to pour drinks because the weight of the pitcher will be too much for my weak hand to bear. I'm convinced that good things are coming, I just hope God gives me the fortitude to recognize them when they happen.

> **BELIEVE IT OR NOT, ONE OF MY BIGGEST FEARS NOW IS CHANGING MEDICATION, MAINLY BECAUSE IT DISORIENTS ME AND TAKES SEVERAL WEEKS TO GET USED TO.**

How am I coping with PD today?

At the time of this writing, I'm eight months in and don't have any debilitating symptoms that prevent me from functioning yet. So, while I'm aware that disease progression may make things difficult for me in the future, I have learned how to deal with my current symptoms. It's been a balancing act between exercise, stress control and timing of medication intake. I feel good when I wake up in the morning but as the day goes on, I notice muscle weakness, some rigidity in my neck, slowness of my gait, shakiness in my hand when I'm nervous or anxious about something, and

CHAPTER 1 / MY STORY

shakiness in my legs after any type of strenuous lower body activity like jogging or paddle boarding. I'm watching my body every day for signs of physical degradation and waiting for symptoms of disease progression. I constantly wonder if my hand tremor will get worse or if it will eventually just spread to another part of my body. Every time I feel a slight pain, a new twitch or muscle fatigue, I wonder if its PD, or something else. It has put me into an altered reality where I'm always thinking of PD and as much as I wish I could just forget about it, I'm always reminded that the disease is there.

What medications am I taking?

One of the things that initially scared me about PD was that I was going to be on medication for the rest of my life and that I may have to contend with dyskinesia. Believe it or not, one of my biggest fears now is changing medication, mainly because it disorients me and takes several weeks to get used to. However, I'm currently taking 75MG of L-Dopa (3 pills) a day plus 1.5MG (6 pills) of Mirapex, which is a dopamine agonist. I also take Magnesium supplements at night before going to sleep and I'm trying a high dosage of B1 to see if it alleviates my tremor. The B1 trial is part of a regimen that I read about called the High Dosage of Thiamin (HDT) Therapy. It's a natural therapy founded by Italian neurologist, Dr. Antonio Costantini and if administered at the right custom corrected dosage, improves fatigue and other symptoms from PD.

What am I doing for exercise?

Imagine if you were given a life changing diagnosis and the doctor told you that the only proven method to slow its progression was exercise. Well, that's what I was told and it's one of the things that I do religiously now. For exercise, I run a ¾ mile just about every day, then I do anywhere from 30-45 push-ups and as many pull ups as I can before my arms give up. Every Monday and Wednesday evening I join my fellow Person with Parkinson's (PWP) Paul Cluff online for a 30-minute High Intensity Interval Training (HIIT) workout. On Saturday mornings, I like to do Stand Up Paddle boarding (SUP) at the beach or intercoastal which is a great upper body workout and balancing exercise. On Saturday afternoons, my wife and I do a 10 mile bike ride and then I run over a bridge which equates to about a mile in distance. Mainly, I try to do enough work to sweat and get myself out of breath because it helps me relax and reduces the uncontrollable movements that occasionally happen when I sleep.

What has been the most difficult thing to accept about Parkinson's?

I think the most difficult aspect for me has been getting acclimated to a disease that I have no control over and learning how to tolerate my symptoms in public. While the medication helps, it doesn't completely eliminate my hand tremor so when I'm nervous, anxious or fatigued, the tremor manifests itself pretty violently. Some days it's so intense that I have to find creative ways to conceal it and it sometimes makes me look awkward. It's a crazy hand dance that changes positions every five minutes or so. I understand the transition into being comfortable with these symptoms will take time and talking to people that have been dealing with similar symptoms has been helpful.

Another thing that's hard for me is the fear that people in my professional circles will consider me to be ineffective in my role as an architect because of PD. Working with YOPD is a little bit like taking a toddler to work. My tremors are unpredictable distractions and my work around is that I have had to teach myself how to use my left hand to draw (using the mouse) because my right (primary) hand either shakes too much or is too weak to function in optimal capacity. I love what I do as an architect. I love solving constructability problems, designing buildings and drafting. Like many other professions, Architecture is a very competitive field and you are judged by your effectiveness at many aspects of the job such as drafting speed, communication skills, presentations, marketing, client interaction, project management, fee and budget maintenance. It's not only a social job but performance based, and any weakness can be construed as a liability.

What advice do I have for someone that has been newly diagnosed with YOPD?

Social media has completely transformed my ability to form relationships with people because all I have to do is send a quick Instant Message (IM) to introduce myself and I have a new PD connection. My one and only piece of advice is to build a network of other People with Young Onset Parkinson's Disease (PWYOPD) that you can confide in, whether it's virtual or physical. Overall, this book has been a cathartic experience for me because I've had to find people, interview them and document their stories, so I've gotten to know them very well. At any time, I can reach out and ask questions or just check-in to see how things are going.

In a funny way, I have developed the opinion that PD has saved my life because its forced me to take advantage of today and let the future take care of itself. Since my diagnosis, I've lost 20 pounds and shifted over to a plant-based diet mainly in an effort to be in the best shape that I can be to fight this disease. If I hadn't received the diagnosis, I'd likely be obsessing about how to position myself for a promotion at work or how to take on more responsibility in various professional organizations. Instead, I'm obsessing about exercise, eating right and engaging with my family. Trust me, this newfound life change has not been easy, but it represents the next chapter of my life and I hope through what you read in this book, you too can prepare for the journey ahead.

Why did I write this book?

When I was first diagnosed, I didn't know where to turn for information. I listened to podcasts from specialists, read books, attended support groups, joined Facebook pages, talked with my physician, but I really just wanted to hear from people my age who were contending with the disease. So I decided to interview other

CHAPTER 1 / MY STORY

YOPWP's to see what it was like to live with Parkinson's.

I have selected these people because in many ways, they are not only living with PD, but thriving. Some are negotiating powerful careers, taking leadership roles in their professional organizations, competing in endurance events, starting foundations, volunteering in their communities, playing team sports, writing books, raising money for research and raising kids. However, what characterizes them the most is what they are not doing, which is sitting around waiting for the disease to consume them. They are finding unique ways to tolerate their symptoms while maintaining hope that their lives don't have to be dictated by PD. Their stories are what reminds me that this disease behaves differently in all of us and it reminds me of how resilient the human spirit is in overcoming adversity, even in the face of insurmountable odds. In the end, I wrote the book because I wanted to collect personal stories from people living with YOPD.

WELCOME TO THE YOPD CLUB

JIMMY CHOI

You were given a life changing diagnosis, so if you don't commit to a lifestyle change than you can't expect your body to keep up with the progression of the disease.

I sat for nearly an hour-and-a-half talking with Jimmy and was completely mesmerized by the wisdom he has gained from 17 years of living with Young Onset Parkinson's Disease (YOPD) coupled with the calm and playful delivery of his message. Having only met him once previously at the beginning of a "Can't Shake Me" workout, I really didn't know him, but he talked to me as if we had been lifelong friends. His attitude was full of peace, hope, optimism and enthusiasm as he talked about his kids, his wife, and the support and inspiration that he gets from his family. At the beginning of the interview, I asked him who his biggest influence was fully expecting him to drop a name like Chuck Norris or Bruce Lee, given Jimmy's passion for exercise and health, but his response just blew me away. "Does it have to be a public figure", he said? "No," I said. "Well in that case, I'd have to say my daughter is my biggest influence." She is 13 years old and has never known her dad without YOPD. I started using exercise and fitness as a treatment when she was about 5 years old, so she's never seen the other side of me, which was the first 8 years of YOPD. To her, I have always been superman and she will never let me back down from anything. As far as she can remember, she has known me to participate in endurance events so anytime a new challenge comes around, she's the first to say, "why can't you do that?" She's the reason that I got onto American Ninja Warrior and quite frankly, it was from a dare. At the time, I was a runner and didn't have the upper body strength to compete so I gave her all the excuses I could think of. However, she never gave up and continues to push me today so, in response to the question, she would be my biggest influence.

For those of you that don't know him, Jimmy Choi is 46-years-old and no stranger to overcoming adversity. Since his diagnosis, he is the second Person with Parkinson's (PWP) to compete but the first to clear obstacles on the famed "American Ninja Warrior" obstacle course. He has participated in countless endurance events but most importantly, he and his wife have raised over $500K for Parkinson's research. After being diagnosed with YOPD at the age of 27, he battled denial and depression for years. He hit rock bottom when he fell down a full flight of stairs while carrying his young son Mason. Thankfully both were physically unharmed, but the fall caused him to shift his mindset and reclaim what YOPD had robbed from him physically, mentally and emotionally. Since then, Jimmy has participated in multiple clinical trials to further research on better treatments and hopefully a cure for Parkinson's Disease (PD). He is a motivational speaker and is active on social media where you can find him competing against the latest "TikTok" challenges in effort to raise PD awareness.

Could you take me through your initial diagnosis?

A lot of people dealing with YOPD don't understand the changes that their body is going through. I certainly didn't and attributed everything that I was feeling to everyday life. Anything that I was feeling: stiffness, rigidity, tremors, loss of balance could be explained away by everyday life. I was only 27 years old when I was diagnosed. I had just gotten married, I played 4 or 5 rounds of golf a week and would always walk and carry my clubs so to be a little stiff and rigid in the mornings and throughout the day wasn't uncommon. I was also an IT guy during the dot com boom and there were a lot of stresses so little twitches could be explained away by anxiety. We can explain away everyday life and not think twice about it. Even when you go to your doctor for a yearly physical, you don't even bring these things up because in your mind, you've already checked it off with everyday life. Furthermore, had the next thing not happened, I probably wouldn't have found out that I had YOPD for another 3 or 4 more years.

When I got married, I went and got life insurance and

they sent out a nurse to do a physical for me. When the nurse was examining me, she began to ask a lot of questions about drugs and alcohol. She said "the reason I asked those questions was to be sure, but the other reason was that I work in a neurologist's office as my day job and I'm seeing things in the way that you move and in your tests that I see regularly in my office." She told me that I should discuss my gait, my arm swing and my pupil dilation with my general practitioner the next time I saw him. She never mentioned the word Parkinson's, but the conversation piqued my curiosity and that started me down the road to my diagnosis.

My general practitioner referred me to a neurologist and after about 3 months of seeing different doctors and specialists who all said they didn't know, I saw my 4th and she said "I think you have Parkinson's and I want you to go see a Movement Disorder Specialist (MDS) to confirm." My initial reaction was, of course, shock because I thought that was a disease for old people. My second reaction was immediately anger and I think I cursed at her when she told me….in fact I may have told her to go F*%# off. Anyways, I didn't believe her at first, so I went into denial. I did go see that MDS and he took one look at me when I walked in and said "Yes, I think you have PD, and this is how we are going to be sure. We are going to put you on medication and if you feel better in two weeks after taking it regularly, you've got PD. It's as simple as that." I thought he was full of shit so I went to another MDS and this was the third person that told me I had PD so I thought that maybe I should try out the medication to see if it works.

To make a long story short, the new MDS gave me Mirapex, a dopamine agonist and I felt better. Over the next 6 months I did a DAT scan twice and it showed changes in my dopamine activity levels which is how I got my confirmation. I was in such denial that I didn't even tell my wife until I decided that the Mirapex worked well enough to take regularly. That was my initial diagnosis story; a collection of all the phases of grief.

What medications are you taking now?

Now it's just Sinemet (L-Dopa). I was on Mirapex for 8 years but the difference between what I did and what you're probably doing is that because I was in such denial, I never adjusted my dosage. I didn't do the things that I was supposed to be doing to ensure that the medication was working optimally for me. I just took it because the doctor gave me a prescription for it and then for 8 years, I never changed my regimen. What happened was that for the first 8 years, I thought that I would take a pill and I'd be fine because I felt fine. However, what was happening was that the disease started to progress, and I was doing the minimal to manage it. I know now that was not the way to approach it. You must be your own advocate and know what is happening to your body as you're taking medication and are doing different things. I never took that into consideration during my first 8 years.

Once I realized that I needed to make a change in my medication, my doctor increased my dose to what he thought it should be based on after 8 years of progression. He increased the Mirapex by 4 times just like that and I started developing gambling and other compulsive habits because I was taking too much. I stopped taking Mirapex after that and started taking Azilect which didn't do much for me. To be honest, it was a pretty rough time because I went from something that I thought was working to the slow realization that this was not getting any better but was getting worse quick which put me into a state of depression and anger.

> **THAT EVENT IN MY LIFE IS ULTIMATELY WHAT JOLTED ME INTO ACTION AND REALLY PUSHED ME TO EDUCATE MYSELF ABOUT THE DISEASE.**

Fast forward to another year or so to 2010 where I was carrying my son and we fell down a flight of stairs. That was my true wake up moment where I realized that I couldn't be a safety hazard to my kids just by holding or playing with them. That event in my life is ultimately what jolted me into action and really pushed me to educate myself about the disease. Up to this point within the first 8 years, I did the absolute minimum and that's just not the way to handle it.

Were you exercising at the time, or was exercise something that you learned about later?

No, up to this point, I was 240 pounds, I was walking with a cane and I was very inactive and unhealthy with my nutrition which meant that I was eating out of convenience. I was still working and traveling so everything I ate was whatever I could get

CHAPTER 2 / JIMMY CHOI

fast. After the fall with my son, I looked around to see what I could do to make a change and I realized that I wasn't smart enough to find a cure or even fund a cure but that I could be part of research. I started enrolling in all the clinical trials that I could find and get approved for. Jumping from one clinical trial to the other was what I did for the next year and a half. I've taken part in clinical trials as simple as just taking surveys to ones that are highly invasive. I actually had three brain surgeries from a clinical trial involving stem cells and my selfish thought process at the time (bear in mind I was still gambling) was that high risk equals high reward so if they find a cure, I would be the first to get it. The worst part was I thought that if a trial that I'm participating in fails and I die, that wouldn't necessarily be the worst thing either. That was my mindset so I was either going to give my body up to find a cure or I was going to die trying and it wouldn't be so bad if I did.

One thing I noticed in just about every trial is that there was always a question on physical activity. I remember one was a forced movement exercise trial where you sit at a table with a physical therapist and they do all the movements for you. I remember coming home after one of the sessions and I felt pretty good by comparison to how I felt going in. Then after the next session, I felt great again and I thought that maybe there was something to this exercise thing. In between the trials I would do the same exercise and movements that they were doing in the trials at home. Then I started to get more active with my family because my kids were becoming toddlers and ultimately when I felt comfortable, I stopped using the cane. The more I did the better I felt and that's when it started to click that maybe there is something to this.

Being the competitive guy that I am, I wanted to see if I could do a little bit better, so I started challenging myself to achieve weekly gains. Ultimately, I gained a lot of confidence in the way that I was walking, and I stopped using my cane. Then I said to myself, why not jog for a bit? I just kept doing that between 2011 and 2012 and I was basically building my base and getting better and better each day, pushing myself to beat the previous weeks achievements. Ultimately those blocks added up to miles and the jogs turned into runs and I started to keep track of how much medication I was taking, when I was taking it, what I ate, when I exercised, what type of exercise I did and how I felt after 30 minutes or an hour. At this time, I also became close to my doctors and the information that I was tracking allowed me to tailor my regimen around my activity. What that information told us was that I should be changing my medication schedule to correspond with the activities that I'm doing, and the timing of my dosing will change based on the activity that I'm doing as well. The idea is to get those peaks and valleys as flat as possible and by doing that 10 years later (I still do it to this day), I'm able to flatten that curve as much as possible. Its tedious work but it is a commitment

> **YOU WERE GIVEN A LIFE CHANGING DIAGNOSIS, SO IF YOU DON'T CHANGE YOUR LIFE, YOU CAN'T EXPECT YOUR SITUATION TO GET ANY BETTER.**

to a lifestyle change. I've met thousands of people with PD and unfortunately very few will dedicate the commitment to doing the things that I do. You were given a life changing diagnosis, so if you don't change your life, you can't expect your situation to get any better. If you don't commit to a lifestyle change, you're not going anywhere. If you're happy watching Netflix all day, eating the same foods that you were eating at initial diagnosis and aren't willing to make a change, then you can't expect your body to make steps in the right direction.

You mentioned having done brain surgeries; have you considered Deep Brain Stimulation (DBS)?

I was supposed to have it done last September and I opted not to because I've gotten myself into another clinical trial that has been pretty good for me. DBS is very invasive, and I would no longer be able to compete on Ninja Warrior because any fall that I take could move the leads that are implanted inside my brain. In July of last year, a Stanford University research professor reached out to me about a pilot program on a device called a Vibrotactile Stimulator. The idea is similar to DBS in that it provides stimulation in the brain, but it is noninvasive in that they are doing it from the outside instead of the inside. This has gone from a pilot program to a clinical trial and the results have been pretty good for most of the people that are taking part in it. I'm right there in the middle range but it has turned back the clock for me to the point where I can put off DBS longer. My doctors agree that I'm moving well, and I've seen a 30% improvement from the pilot program. My Unified Parkinson's Disease Rating Scale (UPDRS) scores off meds was 62/199 before the trial and now off meds, I'm in the low 40's. Before the trial I was taking 16 pills a day and now I'm down to 12 so I decided to hold off on the surgery.

Can everyone succeed as well as you are with PD?

I've been fortunate to have been able to keep myself together for the past 10 years, but a few things have worked well for me and can probably work for others.

The first is speech therapy. Speaking to large groups has always been a part of every job I've had. I was a Chief Technology Officer at a large tech firm before retiring last year and being in that role, I always had to speak to crowds so I've been able to hone my ability to speak and project my voice through many years of professional training. At one point I was having trouble with volume, so I took speech therapy and I practice those drills to this day to make sure that I am projecting, enunciating and putting effort into what I'm about to say. I also have a slight tremor in my ear that makes me scream in order to hear myself. Ultimately, the stars have lined up for me and I'm sure they will for other people.

Another thing is that I also never settle when it comes to exercise and what that means is that I'm always pushing myself. People always come up to me and ask how I do it and when I tell them they say, wow that's a lot. It is and to be honest, that's why I retired so that I can take care of myself full time. A lot

CHAPTER 2 / JIMMY CHOI

of people, especially with Young Onset, don't have the luxury to retire and I get it but the simple question is no matter if you're doing rock steady, or running, or doing High Intensity Interval Training (HIIT), are you pushing yourself to advance? Parkinson's is a progressive disease that's going to get worse over time so if you aren't trying to keep up with progression in your fitness, than you're going to feel the progression of PD. I always say that just because I'm getting stronger doesn't mean that PD isn't there. You're going to have good days and bad days but if you don't push yourself on the good days and take advantage of it, you're missing out on the opportunity to prepare your body to push back on the bad.

I am going to pay a price for this by the way because I can't do it forever. Forget PD for a second, I'm 46 years old and my joints are starting to break down, my muscles ache and eventually I'm going to slow down but now I just need to find other things that can keep me going. This is also a mental game because exercise is the only treatment proven to slow progression so why wouldn't you do it? You can take as many pills as you want but they're only masking the symptoms, they aren't slowing the progression. I don't know if you've read up on it, but neuroplasticity means that you're training new parts of your brain to pick up tasks that other parts are failing at. In a sense, you're creating new neuro pathways to do things and HIIT has been proven to do that for anybody, not just People with Parkinson's (PWP). Your positive mindset also plays a part as well. It sucks to do 1000 burpees at a time and run 26 miles. Nobody wants to do this stuff for fun. I don't do it because I enjoy it but because I want to make sure my body is able to handle whatever PD throws at me, but you must have the positive mindset to achieve it. If you don't have the mental capacity to go into a dark place in your mind and find the grit to tune out the pain in order to just get the job done, you'll never know what it's like to push yourself.

Speaking of marathons and races, how many have you done?

Before my first 5K in 2012, I never ran more than 110' which was about the radius of field that I covered while playing center field at Purdue University. However, between 2012 and last year, I've done one ultra-marathon which is a 50-mile run, 16 marathons, 105 half marathons, countless 5K's, 10K's and triathlons, 2 Ironman's, 8 to 10 Gran Fando's which are 100-mile bike rides. I was also the first person with PD to complete a 100-mile bike ride in under 5 hours which meant that I was holding a 25 MPH average for the entire 100 miles. Last but not least, I've competed 4 times on the show America Ninja Warrior. These are the things that I've been able to do over the past 10 years because of that mentality of trying to get more each day.

> **I DON'T DO IT BECAUSE I ENJOY IT BUT BECAUSE I WANT TO MAKE SURE MY BODY IS ABLE TO HANDLE WHATEVER PD THROWS AT ME, BUT YOU MUST HAVE THE POSITIVE MINDSET TO ACHIEVE IT.**

Tell me about your involvement with the Michael J. Fox Foundation?

As a person with Young Onset in early 2010, I didn't have the resources that are available today. In fact, one of the reasons that I started speaking was to communicate to people that it's OK to go through all the stages of grief, but at some point you will hit acceptance and you'll have to do something about it. The moment of acceptance for me was when I began to fund raise in 2012. I had signed up for my first marathon in Chicago, was new to running and had no idea that 45K people would sign up to run. When I finally committed to it, I was a month away and the event was sold out. I contacted the Michael J. Fox Foundation for the first time thinking that they might have a charity bib and they told me that if I wanted the last one, I was going to have to raise $2K. Now I had never fund raised before so for the first time, I had to tell my story to my friends and family. I had to tell them why I was doing it and what the foundation would be doing with the money that they all worked so hard to donate. In that one month of time before the race, I raised more than $5K and in that same time, I was able to connect with other members of the Michael J. Fox community with or without PD that were just like me. Same age, same mindset, and finally I felt like I wasn't alone in this. I did more in that one month of time than I did in the 8 years since initial onset. For me that was a pivotal moment because fund raising became my why. To this day, my wife and I have raised over $500K for Parkinson's research and while all those marathons were great, we're most proud of the fact that we've been able to raise so much money. If I've helped one person along the way accept their plight with PD than it's all been worthwhile as far as I'm concerned.

Could you tell me about dyskinesia?

It comes and goes and is not painful. It happens when you've taken so much L-dopa that your body moves on its own. I've been taking it for 17 years, but I wouldn't worry about the effects of dyskinesia because everyone reacts to the medication differently. Some people get it as early as a year and a half in and others don't get it until 10 years later. It's about how you process all the synthetic dopamine that's in your system. At the same time, if I wanted to stop moving, I could stop but it requires so much concentration that everything else slows down as well. If I need to speak freely and let my mind think, I can't concentrate on stopping myself. Now remember when I talked about those peaks and valleys? Well when I take my last dose, there is always an over-delivery of synthetic dopamine and that's when dyskinesia kicks in. Then there will be a time when a lot of that synthetic dopamine has been metabolized and I fall into a zone where its optimal for my body. That is exactly the time when I work out and do my videos, but it only makes up of about 40% of my day. Once that synthetic dopamine falls into that optimum level, everything is calm, then when it falls below that point, I hit my "off" period where the tremors come back, the rigidity settles in and dystonia kicks in. Dyskinesia isn't painful in fact I kind of feel like I'm just slow jamming to a song that's in my head. My wife always says, "Oh look, Jimmy's just slow jamming away," and it's not necessarily a bad thing, especially when you're at a stage where you're not self-conscious about your appearance in public. I mean what's worse, sitting there with uncontrollable tremors or having a great time jamming to your own music? The dyskinesia usually goes on for about an hour and a half and then I calm for 40 minutes or so and then everything starts again. Every 3 hours I go through these cycles.

> **I MEAN WHAT'S WORSE, SITTING THERE WITH UNCONTROLLABLE TREMORS OR HAVING A GREAT TIME JAMMING TO YOUR OWN MUSIC?**

Does the dyskinesia go away when you sleep?

Yes. Everything goes away when I sleep.

Has your tremor moved to the other side of your body?

I think it's starting to move to my left side because I'm noticing some of the same symptoms that I originally had on my right but it's still in its infancy. That was another reason why I opted to go with DBS because usually when you do something invasive like that, you want to do both sides instead of one at a time. When I started to feel symptoms on my left, my doctor suggested that we start to think about DBS.

Do you believe that we will see a cure for PD in your lifetime?

I believe that we will see a disease modifying treatment in my lifetime. I don't believe that we will have a cure in the sense of the word "cure." I honestly believe that we will have treatments that will slow or halt the progression of Parkinson's. To reverse it, I think we're still far away because there are still so many things that we don't understand about PD. I also serve on the patient council board of the Michael J. Fox Foundation and we help dictate where part of their money goes as far as research. I see the pipeline and there are a lot of great things that are in the disease modifying category but not much in the realm of a true cure. They are targeting the alpha synuclein, which is a protein that suffocates the brain cells that produce dopamine. If they can prevent these proteins from clumping up and killing the brain cells than it's a win because you're able to stop the progression. Five years ago, there were zero clinical trials classified as "disease modifying." Today there are more than 70 so even if 1% of the trial's hit, that's exciting.

What advice do you have for someone that's just been diagnosed with PD?

The first thing is to give yourself the opportunity to grieve and be pissed. Know that you didn't go out and do something to get PD. However, you also need to educate yourself using trusted sources. Don't go on Facebook asking people for opinions. The

CHAPTER 2 / JIMMY CHOI

most important thing that you can do is to let those in your inner circle in on it. Tell them your story and share everything that you're feeling. Do not be embarrassed by your symptoms and go into isolation because your closest friends and family will support you. I know it's easier said than done but it all starts with education, and not just yourself but making sure that your spouse, your partner, your kids and everyone in your house understands what you do about the disease. My kids can look at me and know when I need to take my medicine and they are 13 and 11. They will help me get up off the chair without me asking and you know what? We must be big boys and accept some help from time to time. Finally, I would say to do the hard work. It's a lifestyle commitment and change.

WELCOME TO THE YOPD CLUB

CHAPTER 3 / LARRY GIFFORD

LARRY GIFFORD

We can't change the diagnosis, but we can empower ourselves to move forward in life and choose how we react to it.

Some people are born advocates. They can listen without judgment and sway opinions without contentious debate. They lead by example and in many cases, debunk the suspicions that they can accomplish major milestones just by grinding it out. Of all the people that I interviewed for this book, Larry Gifford is the closest to changing the world. He is the brains behind PD Avengers, the global organization that aims to eradicate Parkinson's Disease, and his goal is to unite 50 million voices to express the urgency of the situation.

Larry is a 30-year-old veteran in talk radio and is the creator of "When Life Gives You Parkinson's," an autobiographical podcast that depicts his daily experience living with YOPD. When I was first diagnosed with PD, his podcast was one of the few that really set my mind at ease. His playful yet earnest presentation of the picture of PD helped me not only accept my diagnosis but encouraged me to embrace the disease as a "frenemy." He is currently the National Director of Talk Radio for Corus Entertainment in Canada but beyond that and more importantly, he is a storyteller. He has a strong bravado that carries his message over the airwaves and the reporter in him has attacked the disease with an understated curiosity in an effort to share his journey with everyone else. He has had PD for 3 years and is beginning Season 3 of his podcast which will focus on his role as an advocate and a voice for the Parkinson's Community.

Could you tell me about your initial diagnosis?

I was 45 years old when I got the diagnosis, but I had symptoms for 7 or 8 years before then that I didn't know were connected. My gait was off, and people started asking me if I was hurt so I just blew it off. I lost my sense of smell, started bumping into desks and began to lose my sense of overall spatial relation. One day I realized that I wasn't using my right hand to type. It was sitting on the keyboard, but my left hand was doing all the work. At some point, my brain took over and I even stopped taking notes in meetings because my handwriting wasn't legible, and I couldn't keep up. I couldn't throw the Frisbee with my son and I couldn't put my right hand in my front pocket. It wasn't until I noticed a tremor in my hand and pain in my legs that I thought it was time to see a doctor. I thought I was getting old or I was overweight and that they were going to advise me to lose 20 pounds. My doctor initially referred me to a Multiple Sclerosis (MS) Specialist because she thought it was MS, so I saw a neurologist who did all the tests and eventually told me that the good news was that I didn't have MS. I told the neurologist that I felt weaker on my right side and he informed me that it wasn't weakness but slowness and that it might be Parkinson's Disease (PD). He gave me a prescription for Carbidopa-Levodopa (L-Dopa) before I was officially diagnosed and also referred me to a Parkinson's specialist. By the time I saw the specialist, he indicated that my response to the L-Dopa in and of itself told him that I had PD simply because it was working for me. I asked him how we could get a 100% confirmation and he said, "Well, we could do an autopsy - that's about the only way to confirm it." So, I decided to take his word for it.

> I ASKED HIM HOW WE COULD GET A 100% CONFIRMATION AND HE SAID, "WELL, WE COULD DO AN AUTOPSY - THAT'S ABOUT THE ONLY WAY TO CONFIRM IT." SO, I DECIDED TO TAKE HIS WORD FOR IT.

What was your initial response to the diagnosis?

When I heard PD, I was shocked. It wasn't even on my radar. I didn't know if it was a death sentence or what it even meant. That's when the reporter in me started to follow my curiosity and I began searching for podcasts about it. I was searching for a patient centered podcast but all I could find was content from neurologists, researchers, experts and all these high-level people that were ultimately unrelatable to me. I wasn't at that level of knowledge yet. I just wanted to hear from someone who had it and could explain what it was like and what I could expect. I wanted to hear from someone who was going through it, not someone who had studied it. Everyone's journey is different and it's interesting to hear how other people deal with it and how it impacts their lives. Then I woke up one day and thought, well I guess that's my job.

How did the "When Life Gives You Parkinson's" podcast get started?

When I announced it to my staff and went on TV and radio on World Parkinson's Day in 2018, there was a 20-minute audio documentary which ended up being half of the first episode of the podcast. We released it with an article online and people loved it and wanted more. That summer we figured out how we could do it while managing my job. It was exciting for me because I had been doing podcasting for 5 years at that point with my radio consulting company, and I was very comfortable with the medium. I knew I had some distribution points and I wanted to get buy in from some of the organizations around the world because I wanted it to be accessible to everyone. I didn't want it to be exclusive with any one organization and I wanted it to be a platform not only for my stories but for people that I meet along the way. I also wanted it to be authentic to my journey. Season 1 was about the diagnosis and coping with the news. Season 2 was about going from a Person with Parkinson's (PWP) to an advocate.

Season 3 is coming up and will be themed around being a vocal leader in the space and really trying to rally the world to focus on PD.

I'm amazed at how the podcast has changed my life. Its introduced me to people all over the world and its humbling because I get emails from individuals who are starting their own podcasts simply because I have one. They want to tell their stories which is great because the more people that tell their stories, the more awareness we bring to it. I hear from support groups who use the podcast to launch conversations about PD and I didn't even think about that...but it's awesome! More than anything, I was out to help myself and wasn't really thinking about you or anyone else when I started but it's nice that it's helping so many people.

Are you still working?

Yes. I am the National Director of talk radio for a company in Canada called Corus Entertainment where I oversee all their talk radio products across the country. My whole career has been in radio, both in news talk and in sports. I was the first voice of Fox Sports Radio, the program director for the ESPN Network, a reporter, a host and an anchor on news talk and sports for several years. I was the program director in Columbus, Seattle and LA so I've had a very fortunate career.

Have any of your symptoms gotten in the way of your job?

At about 2PM each day is when the exhaustion hits and I take a nap even if I'm at the office. I'm also getting slower at processing and doing things. What used to come naturally, and automatic now takes a couple of hours of work. It's hard for me to judge how long projects are going to take. Details have been so important to me over the years, but I feel like little things are slipping. Lack of sleep really impacts the job as well. I'm still sharp but there are days when typing is an effort. Overall, it's getting harder every day. I used to work ahead of everything but now I'm working to the deadlines.

In reference to work interference, I was having real bad dyskinesia after my trip to the World Parkinson's Congress in Japan after a long flight and time zone changes. I began to jerk while presenting in front of 20 people and they were completely dumbfounded. They knew that I had Parkinson's, but I used it as an opportunity to educate. I told them that I can still talk and do my job, it's just going to look weird and you can ask me questions. When those things happen, I always try to spark up conversations around it. I find that any time other people feel uncomfortable, it's a good learning opportunity.

Can you control your dyskinesia when it happens?

Well when it comes, I just sort of ride it out. You don't know when it's coming, and you don't know how long it's going to stay. I've had episodes that lasted 15 minutes and some that lasted 50. The dyskinesia happens when there is an overload of medication. When there's too much dopamine in your brain, it has to go somewhere because it has to release. When there's too little, the lack of dopamine can create dyskinesia as well because you can't control your movement without dopamine. For me, I've got a good handle on it.

Have you considered Deep Brain Stimulation (DBS)?

I'm in line for it because the L-Dopa works well for my symptoms, but I'm up to the level where surgery is a good option.

What is your regimen today?

I take 16 pills a day and extended release at night. It took them 2 years to get me to the point where my medication was right because they want to slowly build up the L-Dopa. They don't want to give you too much out of the gate because then you will develop dyskinesia. Every time I visited my neurologist, they would increase my L-Dopa because I still wasn't functioning at the level that they wanted me to.

Do you have any experience with dopamine agonists?

No, but that's a huge issue with the PD medical community in that there are differing views on what medication should be taken. Whether it should be L-Dopa or dopamine agonists. The agonists have some wicked compulsive side effects so just be careful. I've heard of people that have gotten hundreds of thousands of dollars in the hole from shopping while on agonists so just be cautious. It's on my list of discussion topics for season three's podcast so look out for it.

What symptoms are you struggling with now?

The biggest thing is neuropathy in my feet. It's a nervous system disorder that creates constant numbness or pain in both feet.

What's been the hardest thing that you've had to deal with as a PWP?

Coming to terms that it's going to be here forever and accepting it, not rejecting it. There are days when I'm slow and rigid and I just have a PD day. I've gotten to point where I realize that I have PD and I remind myself what I have accomplished. I'm the National Director of talk radio, I've got a great family, a great podcast, I'm working with worldwide foundations to help make a difference in the PD community, I'm traveling and I'm mobile.

> **I'VE GOTTEN TO THE POINT WHERE I REALIZE THAT I HAVE PD AND I REMIND MYSELF WHAT I HAVE ACCOMPLISHED.**

There is so much to be grateful for such as high-quality medical care and access to L-Dopa. I'm not a religious guy but I find that my contentment is key to accepting that PD is part of my life. It doesn't define me, but I will leverage it to extinguish it someday. Rather than see myself in a victim mentality, which is how I saw myself in the first 8 months, I call it a "frenemy" because I don't want to fight it and I don't want to see it as an enemy. I prefer to see it as part of what I do, and everyone has something. This is mine.

The other thing that has been hard is figuring out how to overcome my absolute disdain for exercise. Exercise and I have been adversaries since I was 8 years old so this is like a cruel joke from the universe.

What are you doing for exercise?

Finding the time for exercise is tough because I'm so busy with work and my extracurricular activities but I really like circuit training. I'm also finding more and more that my exercise often comes accidentally from my son. Just the other day my son told me about a tree house in the woods that, according to him, was only supposed to be 10 minutes away but, it ended up being a 25 to 30-minute walk in total. It was a cool walk, having to slip through holes in fences and walk through no trespassing signs but I find that my exercise inadvertently comes from him. I also find that it's easier to take a hike through a wilderness where I have to negotiate the terrain rather than on a flat surface. I end up shuffling on flat surfaces rather than walking.

I used to travel a lot before COVID-19, and I started freezing when I approached the metal detector. In general, the reason why anyone freezes is that the brain is giving the direction to move forward but the motor movement is suspended. I have to override my brain by directing it to do something else to get moving like move side to side, or use my toe to initiate movement, or take a step back to move forward. Some people kick a cane to get moving but there are a lot of little tricks to initiate movement.

Do you think the freezing has anything to do with anxiety?

Absolutely. I have nothing to hide from the airport security, but I do believe that its connected to anxiety. When I'm around a lot of people, my symptoms increase quite a bit.

Aside from your neurologist, do you have a care team?

I do have a neuro physiotherapist who works with me one-on-one to assist with my gait. I also consider my pharmacist as part of my team because I see him more than anyone else. You want to make sure that your pharmacist gives you the same type of L-Dopa because they're all made a little bit differently. I also need to work with a speech therapist because I know that my voice volume has decreased over the years. It's gotten so bad that Alexa doesn't even understand me sometimes. I do have a personal counselor that I see as well. I would include my wife, my family and my friends as part of my team too. I've also got an international support group that I can go to at any time of the day or night.

What advice would you give to someone who is newly diagnosed with PD?

It's not going to be as bad as you think. It's not going to be as easy as your neurologist may make it seem, but every day will be different. There are 10 million people that have this diagnosis and we're living each day helping each other out. I encourage you to learn about the disease and find your resources, get second opinions and reach out to your local society or foundation because there's a lot of free information on PD. I have an emergency pack in case I'm incapacitated and have to go to the hospital with a PD card in it. I also have a card in my wallet that says "I have PD" in case I get pulled over at 2PM in the afternoon and the police ask me why I'm shaking. Those are two recommendations that you may want to consider.

For some reason, the instinct is to not tell people when you get diagnosed and I'm not sure why that is. If I had a broken leg, I would tell people that I had a broken leg, or if I had cancer, I would tell people but for whatever reason, we've decided that PD is a stigma. Enough people are aware of the word Parkinson's that they believe they know what it is. But even when asked if they know anyone with PD, they don't. There's not enough knowledge about it.

> **AFTER I STARTED TELLING PEOPLE THAT I HAD PD, I FOUND THE SUPPORT AND LOVE THAT I RECEIVED WAS THE EXACT OPPOSITE OF THE REACTION THAT I THOUGHT I WAS GOING TO GET WHICH WAS RIDICULE, ISOLATION AND SHAME.**

After I started telling people that I had PD, I found the support and love that I received was the exact opposite of the reaction that I thought I was going to get which was ridicule, isolation and shame. For whatever reason, we are ashamed of this and my advice would be don't be ashamed. You've got Parkinson's so Welcome to the Club, lets party.

We can't change the diagnosis, but we can empower ourselves to move forward in life and choose how we react to it. I could have done nothing or told nobody but because I decided to share it with people by telling my story with the media, starting a podcast and now I'm starting a movement called PD Avengers to end Parkinson's. I was inspired by the roadmap presented in the book "Ending Parkinson's Disease, A Prescription for Action" and the movement aims to defeat PD. It's not going to help me necessarily, but I don't want anybody else to go through this so I'm hopeful that it will help the next generation. I'm inspired by the people in the PD community and I feel like my age gives me an advantage to do more and make a difference. My wife asks me why I'm going so hard so fast and I tell her that it's because I feel like I've got limited time to be effective. I've seen other people come through and be advocates for change and their voice is silenced after 5-10 years because of the disease. I feel like time is ticking and I want to inspire and get as many people as I can because it's been around for 200 years and it's time to take care of it.

> **PD AVENGERS IS FOCUSED ON THE FACT THAT WE NEED TO BUILD THE URGENCY, ADVOCATE FOR OURSELVES, MAKE SURE THAT THE RESEARCH COMMUNITY INCLUDES US, AND WE NEED EQUITY ACCESS TO MEDICATION, DOCTORS, WELLNESS CARE, ETC.**

CHAPTER 3 / LARRY GIFFORD

Do you believe that there will be a cure in your lifetime?

I believe that we will find a disease altering treatment that will allow us to live better lives and I believe that we will be able to stop PD in its tracks. I don't know that we'll be able to reverse it, but I do believe ultimately that we will be able to prevent its onset. Is that a cure? It's damn close but it all depends on how you define a cure.

Could you tell me about your involvement with PD Avengers and the Michael J. Fox Foundation?

I am a member of the patient council for the Michael J. Fox Foundation. Additionally, I host the Parkinson's IQ+You events all over the US and moderate the panel discussions. Now I'm hosting their podcasts in addition to my own, I host webinars for them, strategize around media buys and volunteer wherever my expertise can play a role. I also work with Parkinson's Canada who is a sponsor of the podcast. I am not exclusive to any one organization and think that's important because we're all on the same team so there is no need to pick a side.

PD Avengers is about bringing the voices together so we can be heard. If you think of all the people that have PD and all their friends and family and all the organizations locally and nationally. Then add all the people around the world that are impacted by PD, whether they are researchers, neurologists, moms, dads, sisters, brothers, cousins and friends. That makes up tens of millions of people with PD and there are at least 50 million more people that are impacted by it. But the problem is that we're not singing from the same song sheet. I know that we all have different issues, but my goal is to align as many of the organizations around the world together so that in 2024 we can begin to have a united campaign for Parkinson's awareness globally. That way we have the same message at the same time worldwide. I believe that we need to collaborate on research to make it more open science and there needs to be more patient involvement from the very beginning. The patients are not just participants in the research, but we are partners, so we need to be there from the conception to help define success. For example, are we even measuring the right things to determine what will help us? If you ask the Glial Derived Neurotropic Factor (GDNF) participants in Bristol, England how they would define success, 100% of them would say that they simply felt better. It is well documented that there was a huge gap between the scientific findings and the patient experience from receiving GDNF. However, the trial failed because their Unified Parkinson's Disease Rating Scale (UPDRS) scores didn't improve enough.

It's the same thing with improvisation. I started "Improv for PD" with my neurologist's husband who is an improvisation artist here in Vancouver. Northwestern University did a study about PWP doing improvisation and quality of life improved dramatically but the UPDRS scores didn't improve. Well who cares? UPDRS scores are subjective anyways so why can't we measure by the standards of happiness or satisfaction?

The PD avengers has three objectives; We want to get 1 million people around the world signed up at PD Avengers.com so we can go to congress or National Institute of Health (NIH) or the World Health Organization (WHO) and say listen: we have a million people here lined up and there's a million more coming. We need to focus on PD. It's the fastest growing neurological condition in the world. It's the 14th leading cause of death in the USA yet every neurologist you encounter will tell you that you don't die from PD, you die with PD. We may not die from PD directly but we're going to die from complications associated with PD like choking to death, falling down some stairs or from pneumonia so we need to stop messaging the public that it's not a big deal. There are over 40 different symptoms that you can get because PD is a struggle.

We want to give hope to the PD community, but we also need to be real with the public, lawmakers and the people that are funding research to let them know that this is a serious issue and we are silently suffering a long, painful death. I know that sounds dramatic but there are two messages there and the problem is that they have crossed. Now everybody is getting the hope message, but PD is out of control. PD Avengers is focused on the fact that we need to build the urgency, advocate for ourselves, make sure that the research community includes us, and we need equity access to medication, doctors and wellness care.

Our mission is to end PD and it's really a think global-act local organization. We're not raising money, we are not a charity, we are a PD action committee and the first part is to get people to sign up and lend their voice. The only obligation you have is to say yes, I think ending PD is a good idea. That's it.

What was it like to go public with your diagnosis?

For me it was cathartic because I'm not hiding anything. I've put it all on the podcast and I think that's key for it to be effective. I think the reason that people respond to it is because it's not bullshit. It shows the good, the bad and the ugly. My wife and I have real conversations about what's going on. We've been married for 20 years and our communication has changed to the point that I take things so literally now. She says that she needs to record me because there are large gaps of information missing from my stories that are critical for understanding. I say that because those are real things that people are going through and even though we don't know who, we know it will resonate with someone. Consider the gravity of the "misdiagnosis episode" where Jeanette had been diagnosed with Multiple System Atrophy and was told that she had 2 years left to live. Myself and others suggested she see a Movement Disorder Specialist. She did and it turns out she was misdiagnosed as MSA. The point is that if you don't tell people, they can't help you and it's OK for people to help you. She's got her life back now but what if she hadn't gone? Would she have willed herself to death?

> **THE POINT IS THAT IF YOU DON'T TELL PEOPLE, THEY CAN'T HELP YOU AND IT'S OK FOR PEOPLE TO HELP YOU.**

CHAPTER 3 / LARRY GIFFORD

Stories like that blow my mind but it's one of the most popular episodes because misdiagnosis is extremely common with PD and people need to hear those stories.

I've had to learn to laugh at it. I break things from time to time and when it happens, I just laugh it off and blame it on my Parkinson's and then I use it as an education opportunity. I was in a cab just the other day and the driver asked where I was headed, and I told him I was going to get a massage. He asked if it was for physical therapy and I said, no I've got PD and I get rigid, so the massage helps me loosen up. He says, "Parkinson's - that's a brain disease...right?" I think that the more we talk about it, the less taboo it is and the less of a stigma it is.

My family is very supportive and that is important in accepting and dealing with it. My wife is my rock and both my son and wife are there to keep me in check so I don't know if I could do it without them. We don't talk about that enough, but our partners and immediate family see the little nuances that define the slow progression of the disease. My wife is there when I smack the night table with full power or when I punch the pillow at night because I'm actively dreaming about something. Its real and I feel very fortunate to have such a strong support group around me.

Parkinson's has been a huge opportunity to meet a community that is funny, bright, motivated and rewarding. The disease affects an estimated 7 to 10 million people worldwide so our community certainly has the volume to organize and affect change for current and future generations. Ultimately, we have to take advantage of opportunities to educate the public and increase awareness of the disease which is something I'm hoping to build upon with the various advocacy domains with which I'm involved with.

CHAPTER 4 / KRISTEN GRAY

KRISTEN GRAY

It's all in your attitude.

Before I met Kristen, I knew of her as the "whipper-snapper" who runs Rock Steady Boxing (RSB) in Jacksonville, FL, and she is exactly as one would imagine a boxing coach to be - full of strength, perseverance and unafraid of challenges. The written word won't do her any justice because she is such an extroverted, animated and vibrant personality that will not let her life be dictated by another force, let alone a progressive disease like Parkinson's.

One of the main reasons I asked her to share her story for this book was that I wanted to capture her "lightning" but realistically in order to appreciate her energy, you should meet her in person. Her positive attitude is infectious and it's hard not to feel a sense of encouragement when she talks. She is a former speech therapist and has built a Parkinson's Disease (PD) attack strategy that hinges on empathy for others as well as daily appreciation.

Kristen was diagnosed a few weeks shy of her 43 birthday and at the time of this writing, is 48 years old. However, you wouldn't know that she's had PD for 5 years by looking at her because aside from a slight tremor in her hand, she has no noticeable symptoms. In her words, the diagnosis gave her the license to "take control" of her life. She was living in Atlanta at the time and within 6 months of diagnosis, decided to quit her job and move to Ponte Vedra Beach, Florida, a location that she and her family vacationed to each year. She recalls that the first half of her life was spent on the hamster wheel of Atlanta where everyone knew her as a speech therapist, but the next chapter would be spent in Ponte Vedra where everyone would know her as a Person with Parkinson's (PWP).

Tell me about your initial diagnosis

My first symptom was some twitching in my finger that I noticed while driving my girls to school, and it happened so infrequently that I ignored it. I also noticed that I was tired all the time but attributed the fatigue to lack of exercise and brushed it off thinking that it was just a symptom of being a 40 year old working mom. Initially, I thought that I had a vitamin deficiency so went to see my internal medicine doctor and the more questions the doctor asked about the tremor, the more I realized that they were seeds being planted in my mind that it was something worse. No one in my family had PD so I was hopeful that with corrective action, the symptoms would eventually subside. Soon after however, I noticed a twitch in my left toe as I was struggling to type a report and paused. With a twitch on the same side of my body as the growing tremor in my hand, I knew this was something, not nothing.

As a health professional comfortable with neurological disorders, I was suspect of PD but went in to my first appointment open minded. Shortly after my initial consultation, the neurologist said to me, "I've been trying to talk myself out of this for the past 30 minutes but...I think you have Parkinson's. However, I want you to have an MRI to rule out a brain tremor. Do you want to do it today? Yes," I emphatically said. I remember immediately breaking into tears because of the sheer gravity of the news and no one can ever prepare themselves to hear those words from a doctor. My initial thought after being presented with the MRI option was that it was my way of trying to control the situation. I had worked in brain trauma for years and knew that the tumor didn't likely have the longevity of Parkinson's. Waiting for the MRI, I remember being overcome with a tremendous sense of sadness because I knew that whether it was a tumor or a progressive disease, I was going to have to share this life changing news with the people that I loved. I knew that it would not only impact my life, but the life of everyone around me. My parents

> **SHORTLY AFTER MY INITIAL CONSULTATION, THE NEUROLOGIST SAID TO ME, "I'VE BEEN TRYING TO TALK MYSELF OUT OF THIS FOR THE PAST 30 MINUTES BUT...I THINK YOU HAVE PARKINSON'S."**

didn't know anything, and I was worried that my future would be a burden on my husband and my family. I knew that the news ultimately had the potential to change everyone's life, and not in a positive way. As tears rolled down my face, I lay in the MRI tunnel, praying for Parkinson's.

What were your biggest fears at diagnosis?

My biggest two fears at diagnosis were losing control, that something else was going to rob me of my choices in life. However, it was the Fear of Missing Out (FOMO) that I was most sensitive to. At the time of my diagnosis, my kids were 8 and 10 years old and not only did I not want to miss out on their lives, but I didn't want to be an embarrassment or a burden to them as they grew older and the disease got worse over the years.

After having two general neurologists tell me that I likely had PD, I went through an 8-week period of darkness. As part of the evaluation process, one neurologist prescribed a single dose of Carbidopa-Levodopa (L-Dopa) and said, "if this makes you feel better, then you have Parkinson's." I remember standing in my kitchen with my husband, looking at that one pill in the palm of my hand and being afraid to take it, but I did. Within 20 minutes, I felt like stiffness I didn't even know I had was melting away from my hand and arm. There was no more denying the diagnosis. I went to a support group and found myself surrounded by people in walkers and wheelchairs that were much older than I was, and unable to handle the weight of the situation, I just left. At one point, I woke up in the middle of the night in tears and by the time I found the words I realized that again, I had to have some sense of control over this. By the time I saw my first Movement Disorder Specialist (MDS), I had moved through the darkness, had cut back my hours at work and had accepted the diagnosis, but felt a sense of urgency to learn all I could to help me navigate this new path. The MDS spent a lot of time describing the medication options to me, the importance of exercise and from that point forward, I was determined that "we were going to figure it out."

Did you immediately begin a drug regimen?

Yes. The MDS prescribed a dopamine agonist to help ease the tremor and slight rigidity on my left side.

What are your thoughts on L-Dopa?

It's the wonder drug and the only medication that we know helps us function the best we can. There is a percentage of people who are likely to develop dyskinetic behavior as a side effect of the L-Dopa. In talking with my physicians, I understand that a person with Young Onset may want to try and use these other medications as long as they can and then when those medications aren't working as well, start trickling in the L-Dopa to get the benefit of both. If I start taking it now, will it work 20 years from now?

What was it like for you to go public with the diagnosis?

I remember that once I started to let people know that I had PD, doors began to open which inadvertently inspired me to share the news more. I realized that it wasn't like I had gotten a bad tattoo, but that it was something I had no control over. The more I talked about it with friends and family, my path forward started to become more apparent and new opportunities would present themselves. There are so many positives that can come out of those conversations about the diagnosis. I eventually got to the point where others commended me for being open and taking on the challenge of living with PD. Once you accept it, you realize that there are things that are out of your control and that you aren't invincible. My husband calls it an "unfortunate blessing" in that once I gave myself permission to accept the news and make the change, it redefined my purpose in life and allowed me to appreciate things more. So, while this diagnosis has changed my life and the lives of those in my family, most have been positive changes and I am determined to keep it that way.

> MY HUSBAND CALLS IT AN "UNFORTUNATE BLESSING" IN THAT ONCE I GAVE MYSELF PERMISSION TO ACCEPT THE NEWS AND MAKE THE CHANGE, IT REDEFNED MY PURPOSE IN LIFE AND ALLOWED ME TO APPRECIATE THINGS MORE.

Have you noticed any changes to your symptoms since you started exercising?

It is well known that exercise stimulates those areas that are known to be weakness in PD and we are so fortunate to know that exercise works for us. I've seen people in Rock Steady go from a wheelchair to a cane because of exercise. One of its advantages is that it offers an immediate effect with long lasting benefits, and I believe that my regimen of high intensity boxing combined with walking, yoga and tai chi has helped limit disease progression over the past 5 years. It's a life preserver in this ocean of negativity and I feel stronger physically, mentally and emotionally because of exercise. Within the first 20 minutes, I feel loose, happiness and I know that the endorphins are being released in my mind, but not every day is easy. Some days are a struggle to get to the gym due to fatigue but the one thing that moves me to action is the opportunity to see the other boxers with Parkinson's. We are a family, supporting one another through the ups and downs. Some are nearly twice my age and struggle to put their shirts on because of muscle rigidity; others can't walk without assistance. As a person with Young Onset, I feel a charge to be the loud voice for those that can only whisper, the cheerleader for those who need to be pushed or those that simply need encouragement to fight back. Rock Steady has given me the opportunity to not only help myself,

> **AS A PERSON WITH YOUNG ONSET, I FEEL A CHARGE TO BE THE LOUD VOICE FOR THOSE THAT CAN ONLY WHISPER, THE CHEERLEADER FOR THOSE WHO NEED TO BE PUSHED OR THOSE THAT SIMPLY NEED ENCOURAGEMENT TO FIGHT BACK.**

but meet other people that I wouldn't otherwise have gotten to meet because of this journey.

Is there any exercise in particular that you feel is better for slowing the progression of PD?

Whatever you can commit to doing that will make you sweat. Research indicates that "forced intense exercise" makes the biggest impact on the disease. Routine is imperative, so finding something you enjoy is critical.

How did you get into Rock Steady Boxing?

Social media. In my desire to learn more and connect with others, I went to private Facebook pages for those with YOPD. While I tried to ignore the notes of those struggling, I honed in on the posts describing positive outcomes with exercise and saw Rock Steady Boxing was mentioned multiple times. Eager to experience similar positive results of my fellow PWP from around the globe, I went to the RSB Headquarters website for more inspiration. The website offers to search for the closest RSB class near your zip code. When I entered mine, I was thrilled to see one pop up, but realized it was over an hour away. How could we not have one in our big city? Knowing the unfortunate prevalence of Parkinson's, I figured I wasn't the only one in this city that could benefit from this program, so I decided to explore how to establish our own affiliate. In just over 6 weeks, I networked to find a gym, a wonderful trainer, Nate Campbell, who is also a former 3-time Lightweight

CHAPTER 4 / KRISTEN GRAY

World Champion Boxer, and raised $12k from beloved family and friends to kickstart our program!

Do you have a new perspective on the prognosis now that you've been living with PD for 5 years?

I lost my mom to cancer when she was 28 years old and one of the blessings of her passing was that it gave me a new appreciation for life after 28. I admit that some mornings are plagued with stiffness and rigidity, but I remind myself that it could be worse. My oldest daughter calls it "my speed bump" because it makes me slow down a little bit so I can enjoy life a little more. I tell my kids that challenges are an opportunity for you to grow. The more you try, the more your brain can grow. I feel that I'm a better person with PD. I've grown in my faith, my family, my confidence, and I want to be a leader in the PD community here in Jacksonville. I need to be this way for my kids because instead of circling the drain, I'm lifting myself up. This is where the true grit comes from; when you are forced to dig deeper, you figure out who you really are.

Have you found any other coping mechanisms for your symptoms?

I sleep with a 15-pound weighted blanket that helps me relax and feel comfortable when I sleep - it's like being swaddled. Also, for me, staying away from gluten and dairy seems to reduce my tremor. I also supplement my diet with zinc, D3, Magnesium and B1 each day at the suggestion of a friend who is studying functional medicine. Acupuncture is my latest love – I would've never believed that having over 20 needles in my scalp and body could be so relaxing, but it's true. It has a calming effect on me, reducing my anxiety, tremor and rigidity.

Have you considered Deep Brain Stimulation (DBS)?

After I was first diagnosed, one of my neurologists suggested I would possibly need DBS in 10 years, but brain surgery just isn't in my life plan. I worked in neuro for about 10 years and the surgery honestly scares me right now. They tell you not to wait too long because the more you wait, the more nerve cells have died and it only keeps you at your best, whatever that happens to be at that time. It can be done to one side of the body or both and most people feel like it gives them a second wind. One of the downfalls though is that when the battery runs out, you must have another procedure. My healthy denial is that they will come up with something else before I really need it.

Do you have a care team and if so, who is on it?

I truly believe in my doctor's model for the wellness for people with PD. Under their model, you see not only the neurologist, but you see the speech therapist, occupational therapist and the physical therapist every year just like you see the dentist. Because you have a progressive disease, you want to catch any changes in the early stages. Typically, health care catches you after you fall but you need the care team to catch weaknesses and prevent things from getting to that point. The other aspect of the care team is one of support. Maintaining wellness and living with the disease is having people with whom you can share your ups and downs. You have a progressive disease so having a care team in place should be part of the medical plan.

What advice would you give to a newly diagnosed PWP?

I would say that knowledge is power and the only way you'll get to the other side is to empower yourself with knowledge from a variety of resources. I think you have to cast a wide net by going to several different doctors, read lots of books and research articles from different perspectives. You want to have a relationship with your neurologist and feel as if you can talk to him or her. Allow yourself to grieve but remember that while there are losses, there will be gains. We also have to be open minded. The ones that are living with PD are figuring things out and because of that, I encourage them to be open and have a network to share ideas with. Empower yourself with knowledge, be open minded to new ideas, always listen to your body, be kind to yourself, and live for today.

> THE ONES THAT ARE LIVING WITH PD ARE FIGURING THINGS OUT AND BECAUSE OF THAT, I ENCOURAGE THEM TO BE OPEN AND HAVE A NETWORK TO SHARE IDEAS WITH.

WELCOME TO THE YOPD CLUB

CHAPTER 5 / BRET PARKER

BRET PARKER

You have to stay engaged in the world.

I was sitting on the back patio of my Florida home when Bret and I connected on WebEx. It was sunny and the wall of viburnum (neighbor-hater-bushes) behind me completely overtook my computer screen background and Bret's introductory line to me was that "your background looks so real it has to be fake." I say that because having never met Bret before, what impressed me most was how clear his thought process was. He is quick-witted, matter of fact, unapologetic and carries no sense of fear or self-sympathy. He displays absolutely no cognitive erosion, and shows no signs of dyskinetic behavior or brain fog. In short, he's sharp and functioning at a high level. He finishes sentences quickly, even re-words them for better effect, has no trouble connecting thoughts and finding words, speaks with a deep bravado and I can only hope that I'm as sharp as he is when I'm 13 years into PD.

Bret is the Executive Director of the New York City Bar Association. I found Bret while doing research online and knew that I had to meet him because after 13 years with Parkinson's, he is still working a demanding job while navigating symptoms in a semi-public forum. I was curious as to whether the disease had robbed him of his energy and if he shared my same concerns of social distancing when symptomatic, how he was able to overcome the bad days of PD while working a full time job, and how effective he was at carrying a leadership role within a professional organization.

Tell me about your initial diagnosis

I was diagnosed when I was 38 years old and at the time was very early in my symptoms. I had a slight hand tremor that was practically unnoticeable and really, nothing else. At the time of diagnosis, I didn't know anything about Parkinson's Disease (PD) other than that it was an old person's disease and my first question to the neurologist was: "Am I going to die from this?" I couldn't tell you what his response was because I was in such a state of shock from having received the diagnosis, but I do remember that he wasn't super re-assuring. He wasn't a Movement Disorder Specialist (MDS) either so he didn't get into the subtleties of the disease, but he did say that although it wasn't fatal, one could die of complications. Overall, he was very quick about the diagnosis, so I decided to see an MDS who spent more time discussing it with me and although I received the same answer, I felt more

CHAPTER 5 / BRET PARKER

confident in how it was delivered and learned a lot more about the disease and my options. By the time I first noticed the hand tremor to diagnosis, it was about a month or two. Then, over the next four years, rigidity set in on my right side, sleep became more of a problem and I noticed a lack of swing in my right arm while walking. In retrospect, my poor handwriting and loss of smell were both early symptoms, but none of which I thought much about at the time.

What scared you most about your diagnosis and what, if anything, scares you now?

One thing that scared me most was the unpredictability of it. At the time, we (my wife and I) thought of this thing as a ticking time bomb. I knew that I had this "thing" but didn't know how long it would be before I experienced major symptoms. Also, not knowing if I'd be able to continue working, or raise my kids and seeing how bad old people had it was very scary. I didn't go to any Michael J. Fox Foundation events for a couple of years mostly because I didn't want to see myself in the future. I just didn't want to have the shaking and wheelchairs in my vision.

> **THE DISEASE HAS PROGRESSED SO SLOWLY; I'VE GOTTEN 13 MORE YEARS OF WORKING AND TIME WITH MY KIDS TO SEE THEM (ALMOST) GROW UP.**

What scares me now? I'm actually not really scared. The disease has progressed so slowly; I've gotten 13 more years of working and time with my kids to see them (almost) grow up. One of my sons recently finished college and one is in college. I feel as if I've gotten through a good chunk of the stuff that I was worried I would miss so no, I'm not too scared.

Did the disease progress with you in the first year of diagnosis?

No, the first year of diagnosis had almost no visible progression at all. My symptoms were very minor for those first few years.

Did you immediately start a drug regimen?

The only thing I took for the first 4.5 years was Azilect, which is an MAOB inhibitor. After the symptoms gradually started to affect me more, I started to take Carbidopa-Levodopa (L-Dopa). At first, I started with 1/2 pill 3 times a day and over the years I went to 1 pill 3 times day and until about 2.5 years ago, I was taking 5 pills a day (every 3 hours I would take 1 L-Dopa, although over time the intervals between doses got smaller and smaller) and continued to take the Azilect. I alternated between ADVIL PM and Ambien for sleep. (Eventually, I added Melatonin and Trazadone for sleep in place of Ambien and ADVIL PM.)

Did the doctor tell you about the potential side effects of L-Dopa?

Yes, and that's partly why when I was first diagnosed and

CHAPTER 5 / BRET PARKER

my symptoms were so minor, I didn't feel the need to take it. We walked through the options, the side effects, the wearing off, etc. and I learned that some of the other drugs might bring on obsessive compulsive disorders so the feeling at the time was that the Azilect was the right fit for me. I added the L-Dopa first because it was the safest (or at least had the longest track record since people have been using it for decades) and within the first 24 hours of taking it, my rigidity was almost gone. It set back the symptom progression clock about 5 years. I think there's a lot of misunderstanding about L-Dopa and I think some people feel that if you use it too early than it won't work anymore but it doesn't quite work that way. For me, the symptoms were minor and I wanted to take as little medication as I could get away with. However, I was also young and wanted the symptoms to be managed so if the L-Dopa was going to give me better symptom management when I was younger, I'd worry about getting older when I was older. Rytary, which is essentially an extended release version of L-Dopa, works very well for me now (I switched to that from L-Dopa) and there are times when I feel no symptoms, but I can feel when I'm on and off. Exercise helps me feel better, but there are times when my symptoms are bad. I've also tried Inbrija to address off periods that come from wearing off of Rytary, stress and other factors -- sometimes it works, sometimes it doesn't.

Did you get a DAT scan when you were first diagnosed?

No. The real confirmation from my neurologist was that I

responded so well to L-Dopa in that it affected my symptoms right away, so it was clear that I had PD without having a DAT scan.

Have any of your symptoms completely gone away?

There was a point where I would occasionally choke on food or a drink (very rarely, like it was going down the wrong pipe), but it essentially went away as I changed my medication regimen, so I almost never experienced it. No other symptoms have really vanished or diminished.

Has your tremor spread to other parts of your body?

Not really. It's just my right arm and leg and the rigidity is only on my right side. The only thing I really get on both sides of my body is foot cramping.

Does the rigidity on your right side hurt?

Not usually. The only thing that I get that's painful are toe and foot cramps. My toes and feet kind of curl up a little bit and that can be painful. The rigidity that I frequently feel is more like tightness. Because it's brain and not muscle driven, stretching doesn't necessarily relieve the discomfort (although it's generally helpful) so I have to get my brain to be distracted and relaxed. The stretching is good for me, and I need to do it much more, but most of the tools that I have to combat that particular symptom right now are mental.

CHAPTER 5 / BRET PARKER

How has PD affected your professional career?

It's not always perfect and easy. Over the years, my symptoms have gradually gotten worse. I have a tremor and my right side can be pretty stiff at times. I don't sleep well, typing on a keyboard or on a phone can be challenging at times and my handwriting is illegible (even to me) but I've managed to navigate around all of that and still work. For me, work is very satisfying and keeps me engaged and it's better than not working for now. That equilibrium may change at some point but for now it's much better this way.

Are you worried at all that you may not be able to work forever and if so, are you making plans now for the possibility of an early retirement?

I was worried back when I was first diagnosed that I wouldn't be able to work for very long. Now, I'm prepared for the fact that I may not be able to work for as long as I might have without the disease, but I'm already 52 and I don't see myself stopping in the near future. Usually when I talk about this, my wife tells me that if I can run 7 marathons, on 7 continents over 7 straight days, I can keep working. Right now, I have a job with occasional quiet times and many more busy times — I try to manage the busy times and rest up during the quiet ones. I probably can keep working as long as I'm doing it well and enjoying it so I feel pretty fortunate. Part of the reason I didn't tell people at work immediately (that was 2 jobs ago) was because I knew I may have job changes and I didn't want that to be a factor in the hiring process. In fact, after my diagnosis I made one job change and no one knew that I had PD, and when I applied for this current job, I was public about it and I got the job even though I had PD.

Did you experience any different treatment from people when you went public with PD?

For most people, no. Most people appreciated my honesty and were very supportive. A couple of people in my work and personal life had awkward reactions, but I'll always remember how the CEO of one company where I worked was very supportive. When I outed myself, I made it a fund-raising event and he had the company make a generous donation to my "Team Fox" event to support the Michael J. Fox Foundation. Once I started to tell people, they began to confide in me with their various health problems. You sort of become a member of this club of people who have secret diseases, but most people treated me great.

Any reason why you waited 5 years before telling anyone?

Mostly, I didn't want people worrying or feeling sorry for me. I didn't want decisions made about me at work. There was nothing to do and nothing for them to do and my symptoms were so minor that it was unnecessary to really tell anyone. If you have a headache and no one can tell, you don't run around and announce that you have a headache (not that PD is anything as simple as a headache).

Have you ever considered Deep Brain Stimulation (DBS)?

So, when I first heard of DBS I thought: "There's no f*n way that anyone is drilling holes in my head." It's just not going to happen. I don't have enough brains in there to spare and I don't need a drill hitting anything so for me, it was not even an option. I've now known people that have gone through the surgery and some of them have had very good results. The thinking by some is that it may work better for those who are younger or earlier in the disease but right now, the cost/benefit is just not there for me. The medicine is taking care of my symptoms and when they act up, I just work around them. The thought of shaving my head (because it's probably not growing back) and then drilling holes into my skull are not top options for me right now. But I won't say never. If it made sense, I would consider it, but I'll live with the rigidity, tremor and other symptoms for a while.

Do you ever wonder if any of your non-tremor symptoms are simply a consequence of getting old and maybe not related to PD at all?

Absolutely. Fatigue, memory, concentration and executive

function all get worse with age. I've had conversations with my doctors and their views are that I am a high-functioning person so my being sharp and quick helps to offset some of the things that could be from age and from PD. It's tough to tell which is PD and which is the age, but I think that keeping a positive attitude and staying sharp is important. Overall, I have to fight the urge to retreat from being involved in the world.

Do you think that your age gives you any advantage to fight the disease longer?

I think being physically and mentally active keeps you engaged and occupied. The downside is that it may have been better if I didn't have this when I was young so as not to interfere with "young people" activities. But on balance, I think young people tend to have more tools to fight it harder (although I know plenty of older people who are incredible fighters). Some of it you can't control but being young and active gives you a little more to fight it with.

Any specific exercise that you like to do?

I train for marathons, bike rides and triathlons and then I take time off to recuperate. My wife and I did a 100-mile fundraising bike ride last September. This past summer I completed the "calendar club" by biking the number of miles for every day of the month (1 mile on July 1, 5 miles on July 5, etc.) for a total of 496 miles in the month. I know I've got to keep it up and get out there again soon. The low-impact exercise like biking or swimming is better on my joints.

Are you positive about your prognosis over the future?
I feel optimistic but know that because its degenerative, it will get worse. When I first got diagnosed, I didn't know if in a year from then if I'd be able to drive or do anything so to be 13 years later and holding up a busy job, a family and being active, I feel optimistic. I know it's going to get worse, but I feel like it's not going to get worse overnight. When it gets worse, it gets worse … there's not much you can do about it. The drugs that they are coming out with to manage the symptoms are helping me. I participate in observational research studies and there are times when I've had to go off of my medication for the day and it's like my whole body is in shutdown mode which although bad, it is a reassuring reminder to me that the medication works and that as long as I keep taking it, the medication will continue to work for the near future.

What advice would you give to a newly diagnosed YOPD
Have a sense of humor because people can be very uncomfortable when they first hear about it. Most people have a normal reaction to it, but if you make people feel more comfortable about it, they will be more comfortable with you. I also try to be more open about it. It's OK to be a little selfish and take care of yourself when you can. There are days when fatigue will hit me

like a ton of bricks, so I'll take a 15-minute nap on the couch in my office and that's OK. I'm trying not to schedule so tightly because I know that when I do, it brings on my symptoms more often.

Tell me about your involvement with the Michael J. Fox Foundation?

For me it's been fantastic. I quietly reached out to them for involvement opportunities several years ago and have used their website as a resource. I do a Team Fox event each year, support others in their events and co-chair the Patient Council, which has been great for me because I've gotten to meet scientists, researchers and clinicians, as well as the incredible staff at the Foundation and an inspiring group of patients. It's great because I get an inside scoop on how the research is coming, what's in the pipeline and there are a lot of people to talk to. It's really allowed me to help others and although I can't find a cure, I can help others deal with their symptoms, connect with communities and families, and share advice and tips. Being part of the Michael J. Fox foundation makes me feel as If I'm working with a very productive, optimistic family.

What is your Facebook page?

It's called Young Onset PD and it has over 435 members from around the world. It's for patients only in an effort to create a safe and private community where people can talk freely, ask questions and share advice.

CHAPTER 6 / CHRISTINA KORINES

CHRISTINA KORINES

It's like anything else, you get out of it what you put into it.

I saw Christina in my twitter feed one morning in a video for the Parkinson's Disease (PD) Foundation and immediately noticed her electricity. She was sharing her diagnosis story and had some of the same challenges that I did but she was extremely positive, so I knew I had to interview her for this book. After talking with her for 30 minutes, I couldn't believe how much energy she had. At 33, she's currently fighting breast cancer and PD simultaneously but neither phases her because her motto is that "PD and Cancer are tough, but I'm tougher." In her own words, she states that "Honestly, I think that's why I got PD. To spread awareness and positivity and reduce some of the fear that people have around it."

Of all her strengths, what's most impressive about Christina is that she is fearless when it comes to adversity. If I had to describe her to someone, I would say that she is a cross between a big wave surfer and Winston Churchill. Like a big wave surfer, she sees the same mammoth wave-wall of disease and uncertainty that all of us with PD do and as intimidated as she may be, considers it to be nothing more than an obstacle to be tamed. Ultimately, she will break it down piece by piece until it has dissolved on the shore. She's also got a Winston Churchill type of warrior pride who lives by the charge to "Never give in, never, never, never." There are people who are wired to persevere no matter what the cost is, and Christina is one of them.

Talk to me about your diagnosis

I was 22 when I started getting symptoms. I remember driving in the car one day and hearing a weird rattling noise. We pulled the car over to inspect and we discovered that it was me.... my leg was twitching. So, I started to see a string of General Neurologists, each of which told me something different. One said that it was anxiety, another said that it was a benign essential tremor. You know when the doctor tells you something, you believe it.

After giving birth to my first daughter, the tremor in my leg got worse and my husband suggested that I go to a different neurologist under a hypothetical suspicion of Multiple Sclerosis (MS). The neurologist disagreed with MS but thought it might be PD. His exact words were "It's almost like you have PD but if that were the case, you'd be in the Guinness book of world records as

CHAPTER 6 / CHRISTINA KORINES

the youngest person diagnosed with the disease." I then saw 6 other neurologists and every time I gave birth, my symptoms got worse so finally in 2017, I went to a Movement Disorder Specialist (MDS) and as soon as I walked in, he asked me to walk in front of him. He could hear and see me limping and noticed the awkward way that my foot hit the floor so at that point, I knew something was wrong and the tears started flowing. Overall, it took me 11 years from the symptom onset to get officially diagnosed with PD. The hard thing about that 11 years was that I started questioning myself and my sanity. I kept thinking that it was only in my head yet I could feel it when I walked, I was shaking uncontrollably, I couldn't write, I was losing my sense of smell, I limped like a Frankenstein but when a doctor is telling you that its nothing you begin to believe that it's all in your head. I thought I was losing it.

> **OVERALL, IT TOOK ME 11 YEARS FROM THE SYMPTOM ONSET TO GET OFFICIALLY DIAGNOSED WITH PD.**

Sounds like the MDS was the key to getting the diagnosis correct?

Yes. It's critical to see a MDS. I was sent to a psychiatrist who told me at one point that I was having anti-psychotic thoughts and prescribed medication to control it. My first thought was that I don't know how this will eliminate a tremor but again, a doctor is telling me that I am psychotic, so I just went with it. I knew I was giving it too much attention but didn't know any other way to process the info.

What symptoms do you have?

I have tremor in my lower body, not in my hands.

What scared you most about your diagnosis?

My first fear was becoming a burden on my family or an anchor that holds them back. I remember telling my husband that if my condition was too much for him to bear, that I would understand if he wanted to leave. Marriage is a lifelong commitment and I'm happy to say that he's still here. My second fear was that I wouldn't be able to hold my grandkids. I always take those negatives and turn it into my motivation, so instead of questioning my ability to hold my grandkids, I determine that I will be able to hold my grandkids because I'm going to work out and have a healthy lifestyle. Basically, I have become the family motivator and anything that scares us has now become our motivation.

When you receive the diagnosis, you feel as if you've been hit by a bat and people think I'm crazy when I say this, but my life has gotten better since the diagnosis. Granted that I'm cancer free now and I'm excited but I honestly believe that my life started the day they told me that I had PD. My initial reaction was "I got it. We can do this. We'll fix this and beat it." Now I know that I'm not crazy, it's not in my head after all and it has a name, so I'm just determined that I need to work harder. For me, it was a relief and now I had a reason for a solution. When the doctors are telling you that you have these hypothetical diseases that all seem to contradict each other, it's hard to accept but for me, when I heard PD, I thought... "Yah, that I can do so let's just fix this." For me October 6, 2017 was the first day of the rest of my life and I can honestly say that my life is better today than it was then. Every day it gets better and easier. Today is a better day than it was 3 years ago.

Have your symptoms progressed over the past 3 years?

My symptoms have plateaued. My MDS suggested that I start medication at first, but I was against it because at 33 years old, I didn't want to begin a regimen that would ultimately leave me dependent for the rest of my life. Then I noticed a decline in my symptoms where it was hard to move, to walk, to take care of my kids so ultimately a year ago, I started a regimen of Carbidopa-Levodopa (L-Dopa) and most people who see me now, don't realize that I have PD. I've lost my limp, my tremor is manageable, my symptoms today are 100 times better than when I was 22 and overall, I'm living a better quality of life today than I was back then. I think that I'm lucky to have a doctor that knows what's best for my body.

Did the doctor tell you about the long-term side effects of L-Dopa?

He did and he said that eventually I'll plateau and stop

responding to it which is why I initially wanted to push it off. But he assured me that it was so far off in my future that when the time comes, there will be other ways to manage the symptoms. I don't want to lose time now because I'm afraid to max out. I tried other medications but had every side effect that you could imagine so determined that they weren't for me. I was hoping that they would have worked because as I understand it, you can tolerate a lower dosage of L-Dopa longer and it may prolong the effectiveness of the medication over time.

At what point do you bump up your regimen?

That's happened once. I went to my MDS and as soon as he walked into the room, I broke down and complained that it was hard. He responded that the medication should be able to give me a normal quality of life and to trust him. That was the initial start of the L-Dopa, and they began me on a 1/2 pill dosage three times a day. I immediately noticed it in my walk. When I went for my 6-month checkup, he said that I was on a baby dose and recommended that we bump up a little bit because again, I shouldn't be struggling. The regimen that I have now is strictly due to my husband's input and my doctor's effort to optimize the dosage. My doctor takes it upon himself to give me a life without struggle.

I'm impressed with your positive outlook despite the cancer and PD. What's your secret?

I think you have to have one (a positive outlook). My kids are also small, so I don't want them to remember their mom being sad and sick all the time. Even when I found out about cancer, my initial thought was that it was great that we caught it early. I just don't want my kids to think of me as a buzz kill so if there's any motivation for my positive outlook, its them.

Do you exercise regularly and if so, what do you do?

I'm in the middle of active chemotherapy to treat breast cancer which completely sucks the life out of me but before that, I was boxing two or three days a week. I found the best boxing instructor in all of New Jersey and asked him not to hold back because of my condition. We do complete training with mitts and gloves. Boxing is a metaphor for my life right now because I'm fighting my way through an illness, so for me it was important to not go to a group that was specific for people with disabilities because I don't consider myself to be disabled. I work one-on-one with a boxing instructor and he trains me as if I was a competitive fighter. It has improved my eye hand coordination and my cognition as well. According to my trainer, I went from being slow to fast with no current suspicion of PD.

Were you working before PD and if so, how did you cope with your symptoms?

I was a Spanish teacher and I remember that my kids started complaining that they couldn't hear me; and I'm lively and loud so I thought that it was weird. But I also noticed that I had trouble walking to the copier and had dystonia in my wrist. When I was diagnosed, I took all those things into consideration and as much as it was important for me to have independence in my profession, my quality of teaching was being compromised because I was tired of compensating for things that were difficult. They actually had to give me a teachers aid because I fell 3 times while at school, so I decided to stop working. For me, it wasn't a negative and as a family, my husband and I made the decision for me to stay. Being a full time teacher is difficult, being a full time mom is difficult, being a full time teacher and mom is next to impossible when you're healthy but when you have PD, it's even harder. I just wanted to focus my energy on my kids, so I chose to stop working and I was able to get complete social security disability which allowed me to receive the same salary that I received when I was working. I went in front of a judge that granted a decision on the spot because of the severity of my symptoms. Normally you have to wait 3 months for a decision so it's really a testimony to how great our country is that there are so many opportunities to get an income when you need it.

Have you considered Deep Brain Stimulation (DBS)?

No. It's too early in my diagnosis but it is something that I would consider in the future.

CHAPTER 6 / CHRISTINA KORINES

Do you have a care team and if so, how often do you meet with them?
I've taken a hiatus from boxing while on chemotherapy but before that, I met with my personal trainer 2 days a week and my physical therapist on the days that I wasn't training. I see my MDS once every 3 months but could call him at any moment. The other part of my care team that I consider to be just as critical is the Parkinson's Foundation. It's not that they can give me anything physical, but their contacts are awesome. I've done about 40 radio interviews with them and I was the keynote speaker for their gala last May. It was a cool moment because I had my husband and kids on stage with me.

How did you do handle speaking in public? I do that all the time and I notice that lately, my anxiety eats me up to the point where I compensate for my tremor by shifting positions, crossing my arms, holding my arms behind my back, etc.
Well, I don't think that I told you but I'm also taking anxiety medication. That's something important to note is the mental health battle that people don't understand about PD. I have anxiety that will bring me to my knees. As strong as you may think I am, my anxiety could knock the life out of me, so I'm medicated for anxiety and when

> **I THINK THAT SPEAKING IN FRONT OF PEOPLE IS SCARY, BUT PD AND BREAST CANCER IS SCARIER.**

I'm nervous or excited, I start fidgeting. It's exhausting physically, but you can't tell. I think that speaking in front to people is scary, but PD and breast cancer is scarier. At the end of the day. My kids are watching, and they are not going to see an ounce of weakness in me. It sucks and its tough, but you must be tougher.

Does the tremor in your right leg prevent you from driving?

No, I can still drive but I tend to take note of every symptom that I experience so that I can take it back to my care team and determine how to fix it. If I realize that something is getting tough, I will lean on my care team to help me beat it. It's mostly like mind over matter and I don't take no for an answer. I just determine that I'll fight harder to get it back.

I think I know the answer to this but are you optimistic about the future?

Yes. I always say that I have faith in God and science and together, they will figure it out for me. I'm also thankful that I got sick in 2020 because there are constantly new treatments coming out. I have the best doctors and overall there is nothing I can say that scares me about this...nothing.

What advice do you give a newly diagnosed YOPD?

Most importantly, it's not a death sentence; in fact it was the start for the rest of my life. Yes, it's scary but there's so much opportunity and hope left in your life. I think you need to grieve for a second but welcome in the new quality of life that you can have. For me, my life is better today than it was and I'm so grateful for science, doctors and everything that I have. Again, you can live a normal life, albeit it will be different, but its normal. I always say, half the battle is having a positive mindset and a happy attitude. With that, you can do anything. Trust me, if I stayed home and felt bad for myself every day, I would have such a crappy life. I don't feel sorry for myself, I don't want anyone else feeling sorry for me, and I think that such a huge part of living a healthy life is having a healthy outlook.

One other thing that my MDS told me that gave me hope was that with PD, you want it when you are young, and the reason is that the progression is so much slower than in an older person. With us being young, the symptoms and the progression, even as we get older, are still slow so it's almost better to get it when you're young. It's like anything that matters in life; you get out of it what you put into it. Again, half the battle is a positive attitude and with that, you can do anything in life, whether its PD or breast cancer. It could be worse and there's so much to look forward to.

WELCOME TO THE YOPD CLUB

CHAPTER 7 / GAVIN MOGAN

GAVIN MOGAN

Worry less about slowing the disease. Focus more on growing you.

I came across one of Gavin's poems about adaptation and was blown away by how simple the words were yet how compelling and encouraging the message was. The poem reads

Things get harder. So, will you.
The disease will seemingly limit you.
You will expand.
The disease will eventually slow you.
You'll enjoy the journey that much more.
But never worry about tomorrow.
Now is the only time we ever live.

WELCOME TO THE YOPD CLUB

Gavin was diagnosed with Young Onset Parkinson's Disease (YOPD) at the age of 38 and has been living with the disease for 12 years. He is a Certified Trainer in Richardson, Texas, where he offers personal and group training with a focus on helping others battling PD or other health related issues.

As an icebreaker to his chapter, I asked him to write a letter to his 38 year old self to tell him what life will be like with PD, as well as any advice he would give knowing the what he knows now and this is what he said

>I found the cure to Parkinson's today: Stop needing a cure for Parkinson's.
>
>You're going to want to go back to your old self because it's a return to "normalcy" but why be normal in the first place? Allow PD to change you. It is a constantly increasing level of insight into yourself, your life and your mortality. Obsessing to hold on to your old self is the quickest way to depression, anger, decline and you have the ability to get over the difficulty of PD pretty quickly. Something will be Level III hard today and tomorrow it becomes Level IV. It will be hard for about one day and then it will just be normal again. At times things will be immeasurably difficult but you'll acclimate to everything.
>
>I could tell you how important love, or kindness, or resilience is but you already know those things. What

will be important for you to know at the time of your diagnosis is to discover your own truths. You'll find so many answers yourself and the research that you do will be helpful but limiting. As the years pass, you'll find common denominators among people that are living well with Parkinson's. There will be so many differences, paths and circumstances but I think it can be broken down to this one thing: You have to believe that you have some degree of control over your own outcome. Or even better, the knowledge that you have some degree of control. When you have that, you'll have the fuel for everything else. However, among all the great advice for going forward is that you will not likely be ready to process even a fraction of it. Information overload is a real thing.

So here is some advice for you: Engage in things that are difficult and challenge yourself as much as possible because it's the only way to grow. The disease will grow so it only makes sense that you grow at the same rate or more. Spoiler Alert: The possibility to exponentially outgrow the disease is very real.

I'm so tempted to go further, but why? The joy of discovery is at risk. I don't want to take what will be profound remaining pleasures over a lifetime in which other pleasures are slowly plucked away.

You're probably thinking of me as a real son-of-abitch right now. I have the chance to share 12 year's worth of experience and discovered wisdom with you and all you're going to say is go figure it out yourself? Yes. I am and you're welcome.

Consider it a good thing that this is all I have to tell you; that I believe in you, that all I have to say is to relax, have fun, and I look forward to seeing you when you get here!

Now here's the part I've really been looking forward to and you're not going to steal it from me. Go get the basketball because we're going to play one on one and this old man is going to whip your ass! Oh, you can't find the basketball - that's too bad, huh?

The baseball glove and baseball are in the closet. You can't miss them. See you in the front yard in two minutes, wussy. Ha! I don't really to get to say that word now.

The world is out there. Go.

But God will always be in here.

...

At his core, Gavin is an enlightened personality. He is constantly challenging the standards by which we define, understand and even treat PD. What I love most about him is that he looks at everything as an opportunity, learning experience or something playful to experiment with in terms of what the brain with Parkinson's can do. He has a unique ability to use emotionally generating neurochemicals to override his own PD symptoms. What does that mean? It requires being deeply connected to one's emotions and feelings, but it means that he believes a person with PD can use memories, or a pet peeve or a joyful thought to will the body into motion thus completely eradicating bad PD motor symptoms. He has videos online where he goes from a frozen position to running and jumping and his opinion is that he is negotiating the ability to turn symptoms on and off with his brain. The process of understanding his PD is ever fluid and likely grows as he gains more insight today than yesterday. As I write this chapter, Gavin plays on a men's recreational baseball team as a switch hitter so he's obviously having success negotiating the ball and bat.

> **I DIDN'T KNOW MUCH ABOUT PD SO MY BIGGEST CONCERN WAS NOT KNOWING HOW LONG IT WOULD TAKE TO HAVE DEBILITATING SYMPTOMS.**

Can you tell me about your initial diagnosis?

I was surprised to get the diagnosis initially because I thought I had restless leg syndrome. In fact, I didn't think it was something that I needed treatment for so I put off going to the doctor. The only other Parkinson's symptom I had was a little tremor in one of my legs that you could only see when I put my foot up. I used to be a late sleeper but one day I noticed that I was waking up early with an uncomfortable burning sensation, so I knew there was cause for something else. When I finally went to the doctor, the neurologist spent a long time with me prior to delivering the diagnosis of PD. At the time, I didn't know much about PD so my biggest concern was not knowing how long it would take to have debilitating symptoms. My wife was pregnant with my daughter at the time so my first thought was whether I'd be able to hold her or not. When I found out that it wasn't going to affect things like that for years ahead, I was relieved. I just knew that I had to go strong for 18 years as a father for my kids, make money, be a husband for my wife, and battle it for as hard and as long as I could. I had the mindset that "Whatever else happens, happens" and I've always had a pretty strong faith that whatever happens I'll deal with it.

> THE BRAIN PUTS YOU IN A STATE OF FEAR AND LOCKS YOU UP TO KEEP YOU FROM HURTING YOURSELF AND I HAVE TO FIND DIFERENT WAYS AROUND IT.

Did you get a second opinion or a DAT scan?

I got an MRI and they didn't see anything unusual in my brain and after about 6 months, I was able to see an Movement Disorder Specialist (MDS) and she confirmed that it was Parkinson's Disease. At some point, I took Carbidopa-Levodopa (L-Dopa) to target the tremor and it helped so that was an indicator that it was PD. I medicated pretty lightly for the first few years and I had always exercised which I believe helped keep my symptoms at bay.

How fast did the disease progress during the first 5 years of your diagnosis?

I was increasing medication doses every 12 to 18 months. To me that's the biggest indicator of disease progression. The good news is the medication worked well, I loved exercise and PD barely impacted my life.

What symptoms do you have today?

Stiffness like a statue, freezing, some cognitive decline, loss in sense of taste and smell, pain and fatigue. Freezing is the strangest phenomenon and I think I've got it figured out but in short, not only is it a lack of dopamine but it's also the stubbornness of your brain. The brain puts you in a state of fear and locks you up to keep you from hurting yourself and I have to find different ways around it. If I use different neuropathways creating neurochemicals to override the PD symptoms, I can figure out how to move when my brain is telling me not to go anywhere. There is an innate fear that it's going to lock me up. Other symptoms include softened speech and lack of expression in my face.

When you find yourself frozen, how to you get out of it?

Nobody has to push me but at times it can become very difficult and the degree of frozenness depends on how long the medication has been out of my system. As the medication is wearing off, I find that I can move but can tell that it's becoming harder. When it's almost all out of my system, it's a chore to even take a step and I feel like I'm in danger of falling because my balance is off.

What medication have you had success with?

I started on Requip for restless leg and have been on it for the past 11 years. I've also taken L-Dopa and Xadago which extends the life of L-Dopa in your brain.

Have you considered Deep Brain Stimulation?

Yes, I actually had the procedure. DBS has eradicated the little tremor that I had. Usually DBS is considered 5-10 years after diagnosis, but I love it. I'm fascinated by what the brain does under certain conditions and the main reason I got it was that I thought I could cut back on my medication by 50%. The reality was that I was able to cut back by about 25% but the process was great for me. I had a great surgeon and I wasn't nervous about going in. I think the worst part about it was not doing exercise for about 8 weeks after. The DBS is not something that I've had to mess with. I found the proper setting early on and so I haven't had to make any adjustments. I experiment now and then to see if I can find a better setting to improve movement but in talking to my surgeon, she thinks the medication that I was on for so long has habituated my brain so much so that electrical impulses are not that effective. I would recommend DBS for anyone but for me it's been a great tool to have when the medication stops working or if you're struggling with dyskinesia.

CHAPTER 7 / GAVIN MOGAN

Was dyskinesia starting to affect you?

It wasn't so bad that other people noticed but I certainly did. It's like an uncomfortable tensioning throughout your body and it's just distracting enough to affect your speech, give you brain fog, and stressful situations make it worse. A lot of the times, I can exercise the dyskinesia away so it's not anything too severe right now but I certainly feel for people that suffer from it on a regular basis. I'd rather not be able to move than deal with dyskinesia.

What do you do with your time these days?

I used to be a commercial real estate appraiser but the lack of mobility (sitting behind a desk all day) was too hard on my body. It was causing me a lot of pain and stiffness, so I left that job and became a personal trainer about a year ago for People with Parkinson's (PWP). I really enjoy training people and even life coaching but I'm not doing as much as I'd like to primarily because of the COVID-19 mandates. Last week I started up a lawn mowing company mainly because its such therapeutic exercise and I've joined forces with two guys who are my partners in crime. A portion of our proceeds goes to raise money for a project in Uganda which involves getting medicine to PWP because it's not available there. Mowing with others with disabilities and in large part for people with disabilities keeps communities connected and inspired in a time of increased isolation and anxiety.

What has been the most difficult thing about having PD?

Being able to find consistent work and finding someone willing to trust me with work performance. It's hard to get people to trust you with PD.

Have you considered filing for disability?

Oh, this is where the apathy kicks in. The last couple of years, I feel like I've become a candidate for disability, but I hear measurable tales of the process. I would rather generate income through working anyway. But my wife would love to see more of that income and likely sees the real me better than I do.

How did you incorporate exercise into your lifestyle?

Whatever form of training I was doing took on a new purpose, a new energy. I was determined to get better at everything. I took on the mindset of an athlete.

> **THE KEY TO EXERCISE IS TO UNDERSTAND EXERCISE IS ALWAYS MORE THAN JUST EXERCISE.**

It helped that I had two former professional athletes helping in my training. This instruction was invaluable. It made me train harder, but it also made me train smarter. Training was something I'd become addicted to. It was training that I could use off the field or off the court, as well.

The key to exercise is to understand exercise is always more than just exercise. There's so much more to get out of it. You can view it as a form of medicine that can be targeted to meet our needs.

What form of training/exercise do you enjoy most?

The last couple years it's been baseball and basketball. If I can continue to do the sports I love, I believe I can actually get better at them. As a trainer for people with Parkinson's also, I like to think I can modify any sport to meet one's level of capability. Doing something competitive and something you love will push you further than something with which you're just going through the motions.

What are your thoughts on exercise to slow disease progression?

I consider the research in this regard, but I'm not all-consumed with which exercise/training supposedly best slows Parkinson's progression. There is still debate about whether anything can slow disease progression or whether we're just masking symptoms.

I know I have exercised my ass off for years. I've also been decent in following reasonable diet and lifestyle approaches. But when you take me off medicine and turn off my DBS, I would be shockingly incapable of functioning. If I have slowed the progression of the disease, I would hate to think where I would otherwise be with no treatments. But yet properly medicated and with the DBS I am certain that

> SO EVEN IF PARKINSON'S IS BEGINNING TO LIMIT ME IN SOME AREAS, I HAVE DEVELOPED AND GROWN MANY OTHER FACETS THAT PARKINSON'S HASN'T TOUCHED YET.

exercise has provided me with a significantly better quality of life.

There's offensive and defensive-minded thinking:
Defense is slowing the progression of Parkinson's. Defensive is limiting and less creative.

Offensive is anything that grows the progression of you. Offensive is unlimited.

Even if Parkinson's is beginning to limit me in some areas, I have developed and grown many other facets that Parkinson's hasn't touched yet. Thinking offensively allows me to keep widening the gap between PD and me. There's no way Parkinson's can ever outscore me.

Just holding on to what I have will be an intense battle because it always shows Parkinson's gaining on the scoreboard.

Exercise is not the thing that gets you to the thing. Exercise is the thing.

Do you worry about how much exercise is needed to slow the progression of PD?

Not anymore. I mostly just want to be the best I can possibly be. I'm more interested in the progression of me. What do I want to do and what can I achieve? Then, how will I train to accomplish it? Every day I have to work harder than the day before and never want to take anything for granted. Exercise has been my life blood.

What advice would you give someone who is newly diagnosed with PD?

One thing I would say is to take on things that are difficult. Find things that are hard and start to look at those challenges that you can handle because that's what PD is going to be. Over time, things get increasingly harder and the better you are at handling challenges, the better you'll do with the disease. Another piece of advice I would give is to have open lines of communication with your spouse. This disease is usually harder on them than it is on the diagnosed. I shifted my focus from me to her on that day 12 years ago, but too often fail to uphold this conviction. Striking the proper balance between self-care and loved one care is eternal and often conflicting. Also, learn how to embrace your symptoms in public because it is empowering!

Do you feel like your age gives you any advantage to fight the disease longer?

Absolutely, there's more you can do when you're younger. When Parkinson's is your only significant challenge, it's easier.

What is your current attitude toward the prognosis – Are you optimistic?

I take it one day at a time but I'm very positive about the future. Adapting is required but most of what you need on this journey you can find within practicing personal development. Possessing that element of control as other elements inevitably slip away cannot be overstated.

When did you decide to go public with PD?

I went public over the course of about five or six years. I told my bosses and most family immediately. I told close friends over the next couple of years and fewer close friends as symptoms started to become more visible.

Have you done anything personally to raise awareness of PD?

First of all, I realize that I've had access to the best of care to live with Parkinson's and as such, my journey has probably also been easier than most. Any way you cut it, I am a fortunate member of the PD Community, so I am always interested in ways to give back.

Sherryl Klingelhofer began a quiet initiative tackling a big PD problem in Uganda. As in other lesser developed countries, many believe PD to be the result of a curse or witchcraft. Such belief is a significant obstacle to even the most basic care and well-being and the cause struck a chord with me. I visited Uganda in 2019 shortly after learning about the Parkinson's Si Buko program.

That experience changed me. Although the extent of PD in Uganda is not well known, I did personally see many people suffering with it. There is little or no access to the basic medication that so effectively treats this disease for the rest of us. If I felt that this was unconscionable before going, I was adamant about it

CHAPTER 7 / GAVIN MOGAN

upon coming home.

Getting even a few resources into Uganda has helped relieve many people's burden with PD. It is already a difficult country to live well in. Parkinson's is an especially tough add-on because of the stigma, lack of information, and lack of any treatment whatsoever. But the little nonprofit that I have become much more involved with is markedly changing this.

WELCOME TO THE YOPD CLUB

CHAPTER 8 / HEATHER KENNEDY

HEATHER KENNEDY

You have to be comfortable with uncertainty and confident in the core of who you are.

It's hard to compartmentalize Heather into a chapter because she's contributing so much to the Parkinson's Community right now. She is a writer, a film director, an artist, a public speaker, a music aficionado, a mother and a Parkinson's advocate among other things. She blogs as "Kathleen Kiddo" and uses her pen as a metaphorical Hattori Hanzo Katana sword to destroy obstacles in the same way that the character Beatrix Kiddo did in the movie Kill Bill. She is creative, endlessly curious and is excited to learn more in every single moment of every day. Since her diagnosis in 2011, she has collaborated with organizations such as the Davis Phinney Foundation, The Cure Parkinson's Trust and The World Parkinson's Congress. I reached out to her mainly because

I was a big fan of her film "A Mountain at My Gate," which was inadvertently one of my first introductions to YOPD. In the film, Heather presents a bold and fearless autobiographical view of what life looks like as a person with YOPD, tremors and all. It is a subdued and personal piece that depicts the ups and downs of life with PD and illustrates the disconnect between society and the disease in general. I appreciated its candor as I was initially beginning to form a visual of what PD looked like in someone else.

There is an element of unapologetic truth that intrigues me about Heather. Nine years into the disease, she is amazing with words, has a no BS approach to conversation, is literally firing on all cylinders academically and has an empathetic sensibility towards other PWP that struggle to connect socially. She's always hunting for what brings pleasure and is always on the lookout for some great gratitude moment. She has a fun personality, laughs at her own jokes, pivots quickly to keep the conversation rolling and what I liked most about Heather was how easy she was to talk to. Our conversation began with a critical question that had little to do with PD but ultimately set the tone for an ongoing discussion and it was:

First and possibly more important than PD, I know that you are a music aficionado like me so to kick off the conversation, who do you think has had more influence on your life - David Byrne or Grandmaster Flash?

Grandmaster Flash was spinning at a time of unrest and

chaos. It gave disenfranchised restless and potentially lost youth a place to speak their truth and this powered a generation of people. It was subversive - like giving the establishment a kick in the shins when they have hurt you.

More than Grandmaster Flash specifically, it is music from a time and place that I can relate to because this music and such lyrics told stories and proved universal in appeal as beats spread for better or worse into every culture and area. The DJs at that time were scratching records and mashing sounds together and sampling when everyone prior followed the usual templates of making music before.

Grandmaster Flash's influence is not lost on any DJ. Rap and hip-hop used to be street poets that sounded raw end freestyle - unlike highly polished studio sets. I hadn't heard storytelling like this put to beats and sounds of scratching with such transitions before. Though I was too young to grasp any cultural significance, the music and dancing were fresh and improvised.

Just watching dancers show up and spread cardboard on the sidewalk and start spinning with a boombox felt empowering even to observe! As if dance floor could be anywhere. When I saw these dancers and rappers and DJs spinning these lyrical jams, all I could think was that's what I want to do. This must be how kids felt when punk began creating a hyper charged space to unleash certain feelings of rage or express feelings Society deems appropriate for. Some music acts as a refuge, safe but also edgy at times with such chaos and that's exactly how they liked it.

David Byrne is a visionary as well and I've seen him many times but every time he surprises me. I imagine he's easily bored and compelled to try new things. He's incorporated sounds and bands and dancing into productions in ways no one could ever possibly think of... Except him. His voice feels at once fragile and methodical and his transitions tend to be fascinating - you just can't take your eyes off him. He so gracious the way he gives credit to the fellow musicians on his stage, he's more collaborative than egoic and THAT I admire. He likes to sing and act barefoot. The Talking heads were groundbreaking and prolific with projects and some albums for Jerry Harrison and Tom Tom Club with Tina Weymouth.

> **THAT'S WHAT WE LEAVE AS PART OF OUR LEGACY, SO I LOVE TELLING STORIES BECAUSE I LOVE TO HEAR PEOPLE'S STORIES.**

So, these two choices have been fun to sort of compare and this is a great question. One is more within a revolution, but I suppose David is his own revolution! I get incredibly excited about and inspired by artists when something comes up fresh and they remain entirely authentic and playful regardless of what everybody else is doing or saying or what the trends are. Yeah David Byrne is wild and brilliant but both are such influential artists.

Have you always been a writer and if not, why did you start?

Margaret Atwood once said: "In the end, we will all become stories." That's what we leave as part of our legacy, so I love telling stories because I love to hear people's stories. Parkinson's is a weird disease and it's misunderstood, but no one is immune to suffering. I believe that a lot of People with Parkinson's (PWP) are persecuted, which is another thing that compels me to write. After my diagnosis, I just started writing out of a sense of despair. At the time, my marriage had ended, my father was dying, I had friends who had died–so I just started writing and I had no idea that so many people were suffering in similar ways. When you tell people that you have a degenerative, incurable disease, they want to share their grief with you too, because although grief is inherently isolating, it's also one of the universal aspects of our journey through life. Sharing it is one of the only ways for most people to make it bearable.

What were you doing before PD?

I've worked in advertising, I did some recruiting, I've done sales, I was a photographer's assistant, I've worked in art galleries.

Do you still work?

I work in content vetting. I research the footnotes in articles and find out the source behind the source. I've spent a lot of time in the rabbit hole of the internet digging up who paid for what and which editors came from where, who paid them and what their intentions were. Basically, I research the research. And the researchers. .

Tell me about your diagnosis.

I was trying to play my violin and I noticed that the vibrato wasn't working. I couldn't get my hand into the correct position and it was shaking strangely so I thought I had a neck injury from boxing. My left side was really slow, and my trainer used to tell me that I was leaving my left side open, so I knew that something was wrong. It felt like my left side was in slow motion and my right was quick, so I went to see a neurologist.

I was diagnosed in 2011 but I didn't believe it until 2012. The doctor that I had at the time of my diagnosis was a very thorough diagnostician, but he put me on medications that I didn't need, so my entry into the neurological circles was very difficult. I felt like he delayed my diagnosis for about 2 years, and I was afraid to see more doctors after that. I went to several doctors in the year after my diagnosis and was told that I had everything from Lupus to Lyme disease. I finally saw a neurologist who ruled out everything including Wilsons Disease, so I was actually relieved that I had PD because I knew that all the other choices were pretty bad. In fact, I had a party in my head because I was pleased with the diagnosis.

> IN FACT, I HAD A PARTY IN MY HEAD BECAUSE I WAS SO PLEASED WITH THE DIAGNOSIS.

What medications did you take upon initial diagnosis?

I took Amantadine, Carbidopa-Levodopa (L-Dopa) and Mirapex. I never understood Amantadine because I wasn't dyskinetic and still am not.

How did you do with Mirapex?

I did not do well with Mirapex. I'm ADD off the chart as it is, and I think the compulsive nature of that drug was a little too much for me.

What medications are you taking now?

I'm on a neuro patch right now, which I highly recommend because the less you can put through your gut, the better. You can smoke it, inject it or put it in some other way as long as you avoid the gut.

What symptoms are you dealing with now?

I have chronic pain in my shoulders and neck due to dystonia and at times I can barely move. The dystonia turns my hand into a claw and affects my feet as well. Freezing has been a big surprise because it's made me terrified to be in public. When I get stuck it's scary because I'm afraid I wouldn't be able to defend myself if I were left alone. I also have crippling anxiety and depression at times, but I just work through it.

What advice do you have for someone that's been newly diagnosed?

You're in it for the long haul, so just relax, because it's going to be a while. It won't kill you and you're not going to get everyone to understand. The unfortunate part is that this is progressive no matter what we do, it's important to be comfortable with uncertainty. Otherwise you'll be going through constant losses and humiliations. Illness also brings out the worst in people and sometimes they don't have the mental capacity to be around it. It's not that we're needy, it's that we become less flexible because of PD. We become a little bit "high maintenance." PD takes away our capabilities and over time, we feel less worthy of love and the warmth that we receive from relationships. Try not to take things personally. You're going to lose friends; people are going to abandon you and it's going to hurt. The hits are going to come quick at times, so learn to access that one thing that's the eye of your storm (whatever it is that grounds you and gives you strength) and stay connected to that.

Now, the silver lining is that people like to be helpful. So allow them that opportunity. You're going to find in this humility some beautiful parts of yourself that you didn't know existed. When you lose something, you will develop a new talent, and when you start to slow down, you'll notice some cool shit. You have a new family now. Everywhere you go, there is family and our only connection is PD. You don't have to have anything else in common with them but unfortunately, you are family. Have compassion for yourself, stay present, stay in your body. Offer that compassion and generosity

> **YOU'RE GOING TO FIND IN THIS HUMILITY SOME BEAUTIFUL PARTS OF YOURSELF THAT YOU DIDN'T KNOW EXISTED**

to others. Stay connected and try to communicate as best as you can and remember that this affects everyone, not just you. It's confusing and unpredictable and a bit ferocious sometimes despite which, you can and should do your best to enjoy the ride.

WELCOME TO THE YOPD CLUB

CHAPTER 9 / PAUL CLUFF

PAUL CLUFF

PD doesn't' own me—I own PD.

Every Person with Parkinson's (PWP) needs a Paul Cluff to turn to for help. Paul was the first person who made me feel comfortable about having PD and he was also the first to remind me that I wasn't alone. He is endearing and humble yet has a voraciously positive attitude about his prognosis as well as the greater purpose that PD plays in his life. I met Paul virtually on a PD Facebook page within a week after my diagnosis and his first response to my one and only post was: "Welcome to the YOPD club - You're Not Alone." At that point, I was still trying to figure out if there were other people my age who have this disease, so Paul's response was well- timed and reassuring. One of Paul's greatest traits is his empathy for others who are facing this disease and while he is battling it himself, he doesn't let it rob him of the joy of living, working and helping others overcome their own PD related adversities.

Of all the people I've met since diagnosis, Paul is the one that I communicate with every day. I reach out to him when I have questions about medication, symptoms but the most popular reason is to confirm whether my latest ache or pain is PD or old age. He is the CEO of "Can't Shake Me," a foundation that provides financial assistance for exercise classes and equipment to PWP who can't afford it, among other things.

Before we get started, what prompted you to respond to my Facebook posting?

Well, I saw your post and I knew what it felt like to be initially diagnosed and not have anyone to talk or relate to, especially people our age. To me, anyone who is going through what we're going through is like family because only we know what we deal with. People can empathize all they want but no one knows what it feels like, especially at our age. I think a lot of PWP's find it difficult to come out and be open about it and I saw you wanting to connect with people, so I responded.

How long have you had PD and what were you doing before your diagnosis?

I was three months short of my 40th Birthday when I was diagnosed, and I've had it for 3 years. To be honest, my life is not that much different than what it was before. I'm still doing the same things and I'm still very active although I've probably taken exercise to a higher level now because of the benefits that I get from it. I still work full time and I still challenge myself professionally in my career just as I did before. I probably challenge myself more because I'm trying to prove a point. I've always been in high stress positions at work but even after I was diagnosed, I took on a specific position that I knew was going to be even more demanding because I wanted to prove to people that I could excel even with PD. It was a one-year assignment and I wanted to show them that I could deliver a strong job performance with or without the PD label. Overall, three years post diagnosis, I'm still doing everything I was doing before, and the disease hasn't slowed me down.

What was your diagnosis like?

Before I was diagnosed, my neurologist wanted me to try L-dopa to see if it would relieve some of the motor symptoms that I was having such as bradykinesia, dystonia in my right calf and rigidity in my left arm because it wouldn't swing sometimes. However, we had talked about L-Dopa and its primary use as a treatment for PD and part of the reason I didn't want to take

> OVERALL, THREE YEARS POST DIAGNOSIS, I'M STILL DOING EVERYTHING I WAS DOING BEFORE, AND THE DISEASE HASN'T SLOWED ME DOWN

it at first was because I was afraid of hearing the truth. I knew something was going on, but I wasn't ready to face it. I had been going to numerous doctors for a few years before my diagnosis because my fingers were slow at typing and was told that I had carpal tunnel, so they gave me braces, cortisone shots in both of my wrists and physical therapy, none of which worked. So, I finally got an MRI and discovered that I had two herniated discs in my neck that were pushing up against the nerves. The discs actually corresponded directly with the fingers that I was having the most trouble with, so it made sense to me that my neck was the culprit. I finally had double disc replacement and although the pain was gone, the slowness in my hands and fingers was still there. During this time, I went to see my neurologist and although she didn't think I had PD because everyone was focused on the discs in my neck, she wanted me to try the L-Dopa. She told me that if I had a positive reaction to the medication, I'd know what it meant. Within 2 days after taking my first dosage, I felt like a new man and my neurologist told me: "I'm sorry Paul, you have PD."

Did you get a second opinion?

I did not because I knew I had it. When I took the L-dopa and I felt the way I felt, I didn't have to seek out another opinion.

Did you do a DAT scan?

I did not. I know some people live by it, but the scan isn't always accurate. If your dopamine hasn't depleted to red flag levels, it may mislead you into believing that you don't have it when in reality, your levels may not have reached the point of alarm yet.

What scared you most about the diagnosis?

I was scared that I was going to be a younger version of that old person, trembling and hunched over who can't walk or do anything. I was afraid that it was going to happen to me within a matter of a year or two, or less. My wife is great, but I had a fear that she wouldn't accept it and I didn't want to be a burden on her. I was depressed for a couple months after diagnosis and my wife said that I could either cry all day and night about this or I can do something with it. Her challenge made me realize that there was a reason I was given this disease. By embracing it, I have the opportunity to have a positive impact on other people with YOPD.

> **WHAT I'VE LEARNED IS THAT THE DISEASE DOESN'T OWN ME; I OWN THE DISEASE AND I'M NOT GOING TO LET IT HOLD ME BACK. I CAN MAKE A POSITIVE OUT OF A NEGATIVE.**

Was there a point in time when you accepted it?

After about 3 months into my diagnosis, I think I owned it. It didn't mean that it wasn't hard to be awkward in public and it doesn't mean that there are days when I'm not self-conscious about it. What I've learned is that the disease doesn't own me; I own the disease and I'm not going to let it hold me back. I can make a positive out of a negative. The weirdest thing was that a year before my diagnosis, my dad passed away and two months before he passed, he was diagnosed with PD also. It was weird because it was as if he was giving it to me when he passed away so we could share something together. I wish he was here today so we could share that connection even more. To this day and as weird as it sounds, I feel that he's telling me that I'll be OK which has helped me own it more.

How long did you wait before you went public with your diagnosis?

I shared it right away. It took me no time to tell my staff, my supervisors because I wanted people to know about PD and YOPD.

What symptoms do you have now?

I have internal tremors where I feel like I'm shaking in my hands. I also have stiffness in my shoulders, rigidity and dystonia in my neck to the point where I can't turn my head sometimes. You can't always pin the symptoms on PD but when your head is glued to your shoulder for an hour, that's dystonia, not a cramp.

Did you immediately start a medication after diagnosis?

Yes. My first medication was a Neupro patch, which is a dopamine agonist and it has been the best drug for me. I've been on that the whole time and started to take L-dopa a year ago. I made that decision because I can only go so much higher on the Neupro before it maxes out and I knew how I felt when I took the L-dopa before. I also knew physically that I needed the additional boost. I could tell that I was starting to show my symptoms more at work and that it was making it hard for me to work the long hours. I didn't want anyone to question my performance, so I decided to start taking it. For me, it all came down to quality of life. Yes, there is a fear of dyskinesia but it's not a guarantee that I'm going to have it. I'd rather have a better quality of life and get as much enjoyment out of my life now than worry about its potential effects down the road. I also know that Deep Brain Stimulation (DBS) is an option and the technology is improving to the point where it's becoming more and more effective.

What kind of advice would you give to someone who has been newly diagnosed?

Don't give up hope. Yes, you're going to feel that self-pity that we all feel, but you can still have a successful, happy, good life. You have to recognize that every single person has something. Some are more severe than others but we each go through challenges in life. The question is: What are you going to do with it? I would challenge you not to be overcome by fear and to search out other people like you. You need to engage, and I know it's scary, but you have to face it. This disease is not going to kill you, it can only make your life more difficult, but you get to choose how much you'll allow it to control you.

> **YOU HAVE TO RECOGNIZE THAT EVERY SINGLE PERSON HAS SOMETHING.**

When I say don't lose hope, I mean it! When I say you

can still have a successful, happy and good life, I mean that too! But I would also tell the newly diagnosed to prepare for the future. You can have hope and faith that a cure will be found, or a drug developed to stop the progression, while also being realistic that you have an incurable and progressive disease. PWP are like snowflakes; each of us is unique in how we suffer from this disease. You can't compare yourself to another PWP and assume your journey will be the same. However, one thing we all share is that no matter what, the disease will progress and our systems will get worse as time goes on. Be smart and get disability insurance and just Cover Your Ass for the what-if. Live your life to the fullest now, while you are still young and able.

Now how can I say that PD doesn't own me, that I own it when its incurable and progressive? Because I firmly believe that PD can take my body and my mind but it can't take my soul. Your soul is who you really are.

How does your exercise tie into PD?
I don't know if it reverses my symptoms, but it definitely controls them more. Exercise allows me to move my muscles and it has improved my symptoms tremendously. I think it's helped with my cognition as well. I don't know what it's doing in my brain, but I feel it. If I go 2 days without exercise, I'm a hot mess. I only give myself one day off during the week to let my muscles recuperate. If there was any compulsive behavior consequent to the medication, it's probably exercise.

Any exercise that's better for PWP?

I think boxing is great, cycling is huge but really anything that forces you to maintain a strong heart rate for an extended length of time is good. The High Intensity Interval Training (HIIT) stuff is a full body workout that has really done well for me.

Do you feel that your age gives you an advantage to fight the disease longer?

Absolutely. It sounds weird but I'm glad I've got this now instead of when I get older. If I were older, I may feel that my life is over or question what I have to fight for. This disease has gotten me out of my introverted shell so to me it's a blessing so much so that its tattooed all over my body.

Tell me about your foundation, "Can't Shake Me"

My wife and I originally started Can't Shake Me (CSM) with a focus on exercise and providing financial assistance to PWP's who couldn't afford to attend exercise programs. Then about a year ago my wife and our friend Anna and fellow PWP started discussing expanding CSM's focus. Anna and I had always complained about the lack of services for YOPD and awareness of it, so why not use CSM to change this? After discussion with my wife, we decided to change CSM's mission. CSM as it is today is a collaboration between Anna, my wife and me. Our Mission is to increase awareness about Young Onset Parkinson's Disease and provide services specifically designed for this community. Our vision is a world where all those with YOPD have the resources they need to live a fulfilling life beyond their diagnosis. We have consolidated our services into a "Holistic Wellness Network" that offers support in the following areas:

- **Mind**—Educational Programs, Research and Treatment and Financial Planning.
- **Body**—Physical Fitness Classes including YOPD led HIIT Workouts, Boxing and more, Diet and Nutrition advice, etc
- **Community**—Relationships, Life Partner Support, Mentor Program and Social Events

In addition, we've always seen the value in using exercise to slow the progression of the disease so we have created a "Can't Shake Me" YouTube Channel that features 30 minute HIIT workout videos that are tailored for PWP. I've got over 50 subscribers and its growing.

It took a year to get all the paperwork completed for CSM but we became official on January 1, 2020. We are supported by a community grant from the Parkinson's Foundation and had our first fund raiser in February. The second was interrupted by Covid-19. Ultimately, we want CSM to be there when people first find out about their YOPD diagnosis; not only helping them with exercise but also helping to find doctors and medical resources, information on various medications, etc. The website is www.cantshakeme.org and it includes links to exercise videos, a blog, a list of events and much more.

INTRODUCTION TO PAOLA CELI

INTRODUCTION OF PAOLA CELI
BY GAVIN MOGAN

The line to meet Paola Celi was several people deep and I almost went home. A crowd of YOPD attendees had just heard her condense her amazing life story into five minutes. Many people in the room shared their own tough stories; however, none compared to this one. Her Parkinson's experience was one that could add valuable perspective to anyone else's. Finally, just about everyone else had left when I introduced myself. Not long after that meeting I would begin helping Paola document 26 years of Parkinson's in her 38 years of life.

It is extremely rare for onset of PD before age 38, Paola's current age. Termed Juvenile Parkinsonism when diagnosed before 20, instances are so rare, especially among females, that very little research even exists. Paola was diagnosed with Juvenile Parkinsonism over 20 years ago, at the age of 12. Let that sink in.

After about five years many with PD have begun to accept reduced workloads or to retire altogether. Paola was graduating high school and preparing to spend a year-long adventure working and traveling in Europe.

After about 10 years, many with PD have either had deep-brain stimulation surgery to relieve symptoms, are strongly considering the procedure, or are no longer candidates by this time due to advanced age and waning health. They also likely suffer from much more noticeable symptoms. Paola was receiving her degree in Economics from Catholic University.

After about 15 years, many with PD need assistance with walking and other daily functions. Quality of life is significantly impaired. Cognitive and psychological effects are also common at this stage. Paola had recently married and had her first child 15 years after diagnosis.

After about 20 years, most with PD have reached the last stage of the five-stage Parkinson's Scale, likely bedridden or confined to a wheelchair. Perhaps above all, 20 years of Parkinson's damage is grueling on the spirit. Hope and will are critical components in living well with PD. Final stage Parkinson's is an extremely challenging place to maintain optimism. Twenty years after her initial diagnosis, Paola was changing her youngest child's diapers, bonding with neighborhood mothers and their children, and passionately embarking on her home-based business.

Part of maximizing her time is offering encouragement to young women experiencing similar challenges. Paola has only

INTRODUCTION TO PAOLA CELI

within the past year or so began to fully accept her physical state and her probable future. It took about two decades for her to fully accept her diagnosis. Yet she is still only 38 and has a profound wisdom well beyond those years. She believes that there is meaning for the frustration and suffering felt over most of her young life. She knows that there will always be unanswered questions as well.

Paola demonstrates that the mind can be cultivated and intensified well beyond that of any muscle. Minds can even strengthen at a pace that counters physical weakening. Strong minds can lead to desired outcomes. This is her foremost message, confirmed repeatedly in her life. Conviction of mind has enabled a much fuller life than anyone would have expected from that girl 21 years ago. In fact, she has already experienced more of life than many without PD at any age.

Paola conveys authenticity in both her words and actions. Insincerity and trivial matters were eliminated long ago as she continually restructures for efficiency. She may never receive clarity on the meaning of her hardships. However, her path may be invaluable to untold others facing formidable challenges. Invaluable to people awed by perhaps the most inspirational member of the global PD community. Invaluable as a model, and with a message, to those who feel "ordinary" and hunger for that social admiration: Appreciate the joy in the ordinary.

Paola says, "Life with two small children is very hard but I wouldn't change my life for anything. They are my reason to keep fighting. I want so many things for them. That is why I can't regret having PD. I have to try harder, look forward, and move on with hope."

She also may never contemplate the possibility that the most significant, unforeseen side effect of her near-lifelong PD battle is her over-abundant strength and hope absorbed by countless others in their own uphill journeys. Still, every single mind has its limits, even those bathed in optimism. She has faith that the collective mind of medical research will unravel the mysteries of PD.

Paola's hope is that sharing her remarkable journey will resonate with one or more people who are inspired to not only live life to its fullest but perhaps to also put an end to the disease itself, or at least the constant challenges it presents us. This is something that I would love to find out.

Love is limitless. So is my friend Paola Celi.

...

CHAPTER 10 / PAOLA CELI

PAOLA CELI

Life doesn't have to be perfect to be wonderful.

One of the reasons that I wanted to interview Paola for this book is because she had to overcome so many of the adversities associated with PD in very public phases of her life. Most of us don't get diagnosed with YOPD until we are in our mid-thirties or forties and it happens at a time when we've already lived out some or most of our big moments (college, marriage, kids, work). However, she went through these PD challenges before the rest of us so I was curious as to what life was like for her to grow up with Parkinson's Disease.

Can you tell me about your diagnosis?
When I was 12-years-old, I remember having a series of uncanny symptoms that I didn't think much about at the time but

would prove to be the beginning of Parkinson's Disease for me. My handwriting was very small and illegible, I was slow to process my dictations at school, I had trouble buttoning my shirt when getting ready in the morning, my right arm didn't swing when I walked and my foot would turn toward the inside when I walked. What made me feel helpless though was not being able to write numbers. I was really good at math and then one day it was like my brain wasn't sending the message to my hand to write any numbers. So, my mom took me to my grandfather's neurologist for a consultation. My grandfather had Parkinson's so aside from him, I didn't know anything about the disease, and he was unable to take care of himself, so I knew I didn't want to be like that. After multiple scans and MRI's, they diagnosed me with Juvenile Parkinson's Disease.

What was your response to the news?

Well, shock at first because I didn't know anything about the disease and didn't know anyone my age, especially in Ecuador that had it. Bear in mind that this was also 26 years ago so there also wasn't a lot of medications available to treat symptoms. So, I had to accept it, not knowing why it happened to me. Looking back on it now, my parents were going through a divorce and I believe that the stress incurred at that time was partly responsible for my diagnosis so early in life. The doctor immediately put me on Sinemet and a few years later my mother took me to Houston, Texas for a second opinion and to see if there were any other treatments available to manage my symptoms. I went to Baylor College of Medicine and they confirmed the diagnosis so at that point, I was 15 and had been dealing with symptoms for three years.

What was your medication regimen at initial diagnosis?

The neurologist wanted me to start with 1 pill of Sinemet a day but knowing that the disease was degenerative, my mom insisted that I start with 1/2 pill each day. Through trial and error, I ultimately discovered what I could and could not do with the medication. For example, I didn't know that I couldn't take the medication with food or that protein competed with it so for me, those first years was a learning process. Until changing my medication recently I was taking 1/2 pill every 2 hours.

Are you taking Sinemet anymore?

No, and the main reason is that because I'm taking Rytary which allows me to minimize my dosage throughout the day thereby leaving me less dependent on L-Dopa.

Have you taken any medication other than Sinemet?

Yes, I've taken Apexor, Amantadine for dyskinesia, Lexapro, Rytary and Mirapex. I take one Rytary every 4 hours, three Mirapex during the day, and one Lexapro.

How do you like Mirapex?

At the beginning, it made me into a compulsive shopper, but I didn't spend much. I just had to leave my house and go. Now, I'm controlling it and I don't feel the urge as much. Your mind is more powerful than the medication so you can control it.

Some people begin to experience dyskinesia as a side effect of taking Sinemet, but they are much older than you were. Did you experience dyskinesia and if so, how did you cope with it at such a young age?

Yes, I was around 19 years old when I started to experience dyskinesia. Dyskinesia is the side effect of too much dopamine in your body and you may experience involuntary movements like twisting. I remember working at the stock exchange and my boss commented that I was hyperactive because I moved around so much but at the time, I didn't know that it was dyskinesia. The time when I felt most dyskinetic was after I got married and relocated to Texas. At that point, I was going through a major relocation and there were a lot of lifestyle triggers that made my symptoms worse. Today, I only feel dyskinetic when I'm nervous or anxious but sometimes if my doses are too close together, I move around quite a bit.

> **DYSKINESIA IS THE SIDE EFECT OF TOO MUCH DOPAMINE IN YOUR BODY AND YOU MAY EXPERIENCE INVOLUNTARY MOVEMENTS LIKE TWISTING.**

What was life like at such a young age with PD?

I hid my symptoms well, so nobody knew that there was anything wrong with me, and I lived a pretty normal life except for the fact that I took medication. Bear in mind that at a young age, I didn't know that the symptoms were connected to PD.

What was college like with Parkinson's?

College was difficult because I didn't want anyone to know that I had Parkinson's. When I was "off," I would tell my professors that I needed to take blood pressure medication in order to take my tests because I didn't want them to know that I had PD. Sometimes I would ask if I could retake my exams when I felt better. Apart from those moments when I was "off," I managed well. I went out a lot and socialized but I had to have my medication to function properly.

Before I went to college I traveled through Europe. Looking back on it that's probably when I started to develop balancing problems because of the weight of my backpack. I don't have any issues with shaking, but I do have balance problems and I fall a lot. My knees are in bad shape because I use them to prevent myself from falling. When I feel myself falling or losing my balance, I go straight to my knees to stabilize myself and then I push myself off to build momentum so that I can resume my pace. It's kind of like transferring the center of gravity from my chest to my knees so that I can continue moving. Another thing I do to avoid falling is walk on my tip toes to speed up my pace.

Tell me about your life now?

Well, I graduated from college with an economics degree, so I am an economist and spent 4 years on the floor of the Ecuador Stock Exchange Magazine writing articles on market trends. I also love decorating homes, so I got a license as a home stager and I also got my real estate license. I'm also a full-time mother of two boys and a wife so I'm well occupied. I personally believe that staying busy keeps my mind active, so I try to stay occupied as much as possible. When I'm bored, I start moving furniture around and decorating rooms. I never let myself dwell on the disease.

As a Realtor is it difficult to work with the public?

Sometimes, especially when I need to show homes. I try to work with existing clients, but staging is hard because I do everything. I'm the handyman, the mover, the owner and I think that I can do everything. The problem is that I don't know my limits. I'm very strong-minded so I believe that I can do anything if I have the time but when I feel pressure, nothing goes well.

Do you exercise?

When I was in Ecuador, I lost a lot of weight because of my dyskinesias so I started going to the gym hoping to build muscle tone, but it didn't help that much. Honestly, my daily activities are enough for me, so I don't feel like I need to do much exercise. My muscles are constantly exercising by themselves, so I think that Parkinson's inadvertently has made me stronger and helped me push beyond my limits. In all actuality, I'm a frustrated ballerina but my balance won't help me, so I do pole fitness. I have done a spartan race which was very difficult and honestly, I don't know that I could do it again. When I have dyskinesias, my muscles are constantly contracting to control the movement, so I feel like I'm constantly exercising.

What has been the hardest thing to deal with?

Of all the symptoms and years of PD, the hardest thing that I've dealt with is not being fast enough to respond to my kids when they were babies. When my second baby was born, I couldn't change his diaper fast enough and he had terrible diaper rashes. I also think the hormone changes in a woman makes the disease more difficult to bear. I honestly believe that there is a connection between hormones and the disease because when I was pregnant, everything was perfect. I was considered high risk because of my PD but otherwise I had a perfect pregnancy. However, every month when I have my period, my PD symptoms are at their worst. When I gave birth to my sons, I didn't take any medication for the first two days and I thought "Wow, giving birth is a miracle because my PD is gone!" Most of the women with PD are older and don't experience hormone changes anymore so that

> **OF ALL THE SYMPTOMS AND YEARS OF PD, THE HARDEST THING THAT I'VE DEALT WITH IS NOT BEING FAST ENOUGH TO RESPOND TO MY KIDS WHEN THEY WERE BABIES.**

is something that I want to focus on.

Have you considered Deep Brain Stimulation (DBS)?

I considered it a few years ago but decided against it because it won't help with my balance. They said that it really helps with dyskinesia and tremors, but I've been dealing with them for so long that my body knows how to fight it.

How did you meet your husband?

We met at a club in Ecuador and started a long-distance relationship for several months. I was in college at the time and one day he told me that he liked the way I was moving and that I looked active and optimistic. At the 5-month mark, he surprised me by coming to visit on my birthday and I decided that since it was getting serious, that I'd better tell him. I explained everything, and he told me that he didn't care about it, was convinced that we were meant to be together and that he was going to be next to me for help and support. That moment, I knew that he was the one. A year later, we got married and shortly thereafter we moved to Austin.

What advice would you give to someone that's newly diagnosed?

The worst thing that I did for myself was hide my symptoms. It made me feel anxious to think that people would see me differently so my first piece of advice would be to remember that everyone has something whether it be wearing glasses or diabetes. It is a reality that we must face so best to face it looking up and not down because there is nothing to be ashamed of.

My second piece of advice is to not try to be a superhero and pretend that you are perfect. It made me anxious to think that my pills may not work, and that everyone would know that something was wrong with me. I would have panic attacks thinking that if I fell crossing the street, I wouldn't want anyone to help me. I wanted everyone to see me as perfect but we're only human. You have the disease for a purpose, and you were chosen for a reason. The first step in effective treatment is to accept yourself. We think that everyone is watching us, noticing the way we walk or fidget when we're trying to slide the credit card into the machine, but in reality, no one cares. It took me 20 years to accept myself after diagnosis and I finally just accepted that PD is my life, it's part of who I am so there is no reason to cover it up. Acceptance has made me stronger.

> **IT IS A REALITY THAT WE MUST FACE SO BEST TO FACE IT LOOKING UP AND NOT DOWN BECAUSE THERE IS NOTHING TO BE ASHAMED OF.**

After 26 years of PD, how do you maintain your sanity and remain positive?

I think everyone has the ability, but some people haven't discovered it yet. Even though we have PD, we are perfect anyways. Parkinson's doesn't make us any less of ourselves, we just must find our new normal. I know we have bad days and good but most of the days are good. Our life is like a book. We'll have good chapters and bad. Each chapter will close, and we'll start new ones but together they will read as a best seller. Life doesn't need to be perfect to be wonderful.

What's next for you?

I try to focus on my today and not worry so much about the future. I want to be successful within my limits. So far, I'm personally and professionally successful but now I want to help other people like me to live well with the disease.

CLOSING REMARKS

BY CHRISTIAN HAGESETH, M.D.

So, you have been diagnosed with an incurable, irreversible, progressive, degenerative disease of the brain called Parkinson's disease (PD). When neurologists first tell you that, their voices drop in pitch and they may look you in the eye for the first time in the interview. "I'm sorry to tell you that you have Parkinson's disease. While it is an incurable and degenerative disease, we do have some medications that will partially block some of your symptoms for a time. Later, there is brain surgery that can make a significant improvement in some symptoms, but we resort to that only when your medications have stopped working."

Too often, the Person with Parkinson's (PWP) leaves that visit confused with scores of unanswered questions swirling around in his or her head. Even many PD organizations that have been established to guide PWPs to the most healthy lifestyles dwell first on how difficult simple things like buttoning your shirt or eating with utensils may become.

A year after I was diagnosed, when my motor symptoms weren't so bad, I ran into an old friend. Ten years had elapsed since the last time we saw each other. When, in the course of catching up, I told her I had PD, her eyes filled with tears and she repeated, "I'm so sorry; I am so very sorry."

What is the result of all this doom and gloom? Despair and hopelessness.

I directed our support program in northern Colorado for six years. Several times the newly-diagnosed attendees were near tears for most of their first meeting, physically wringing their hands. But our meetings were intentionally upbeat and positive. At the end of a meeting, I would get a couple of our most optimistic PWPs to corner the newbies and we would demonstrate how well we were doing. The following month the newbies returned smiling, bright, and laughing.

What happened? They shifted their mindsets.

What I have witnessed in medicine today is a pervasive lack of appreciation of how the power of mind can alter the course of PD for the better. Sadly, many mid-stage PWPs adopt a preoccupation with meds, meds, and more meds. That is putting the wrong information into the mind. Always, your focus needs to be on what you can do with your Body-Mind. That should be at the forefront of your thinking. Let the neurologists fuss over meds;

CLOSING REMARKS

they have trained long and hard to do so.

When I look at the broad scope of illnesses that can afflict us from the middle of our lives onward, PD isn't all that bad. Consider brittle insulin-dependent diabetes, rheumatoid arthritis, any of several autoimmune diseases (such as lupus)—even worse, severe depressive disease that urges taking one's own life to finally be free.

No, in my humble opinion, PD isn't as bad as a host of diseases that can rob you of a meaningful life. I've had symptoms of PD for over fifteen years; first motor symptoms started nine years ago. I started meds three months ago. I'm only taking one or two Sinemet a day.

This quote from Hippocrates, the father of modern medicine, forms the basis of my thinking:

"Don't tell me what disease the patient has;
tell me instead what patient has the disease."

The ominous predictions of PD's downhill course come from lumping all PWPs together as if we're all alike. But that's a fallacy; we may have the same disease; but how it affects us is unique to each of us.

What accounts for our becoming outliers? How we manage our minds. How do we accomplish that? By changing what we consciously do with our bodies—all the time.

Consider the following:
- Never give in to slouching with your shoulders/chest.
- Stand upright. Correct your posture every waking minute.
- Stand with your back against the wall for five minutes twice a day. Heels, butt, back, and head all touching the wall.
- When just standing in one place, adopt the parade-rest stance from the military. See an example online.
- When you walk, continue the posture you practiced against the wall.
- As you walk, lead with your chest and smile your most confident smile.
- Accentuate your natural arm swing.
- Land with a heel strike.
- Take long strides all the time.
- Get a Fitbit and aim to walk 7500 steps five days a week.
- Learn one of these: Yoga, Tai Chi, or Qi Gong. Practice it five times a week.
- Take up boxing for PD.
- Start resistance training (i.e. weightlifting) with a competent coach.
- Look ahead in life and see yourself becoming stronger every day.
- Limit reading about PD. Once you know the basics, you know enough to be a successful PWP.
- Join a PD support group, but only if it is upbeat.

CLOSING REMARKS

Here are four books you should read to understand the potential of your Body-Mind.

1. "Suggestible You" by Erik Vance
2. "Cure" by Jo Marchant
3. "Optimal Health with PD" by Monique Giroux, Ph.D.
4. "A Laughing Place" by Christian Hageseth, M.D.

    Final words: I have an easier version of PD than you who have with Young Onset Parkinson's Disease, but I hope that my thoughts and advice can help make a huge difference in your life.

WELCOME TO THE YOPD CLUB

ACKNOWLEDGMENTS

I want to thank Paul Cluff for inspiring the title of this book. Paul was the first person with YOPD that I met and his energy and enthusiasm were pivotal at a time in my life when I wasn't sure how to see myself.

I want to thank Christian Hageseth for giving me the initial boost of confidence to believe that I still had a lot of life to live.

I want to thank my son Keenan for reminding me that everyone is dealing with something and for comparing my hand tremor to his red face. You'll never know how reassuring that was for me to hear.

I want to thank my daughter Ava for reminding me that I can do anything if I set my mind to it.

Lastly, I want to thank my wife Kirsten for being my rock during these changing times. I know she didn't sign up for this when she married me and I hope that we can continue to laugh and have fun as this disease progresses and time goes on.

WELCOME TO THE YOPD CLUB

www.ingramcontent.com/pod-product-compliance
Lightning Source LLC
Chambersburg PA
CBHW060839220526
45466CB00003B/1163